Certified Coding Specialist (CCS) Exam Preparation

Tenth Edition

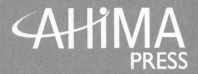

Copyright ©2020 by the American Health Information Management Association. All rights reserved. Except as permitted under the Copyright Act of 1976, no part of this publication may be reproduced, stored in a retrieval system, or transmitted, in any form or by any means, electronic, photocopying, recording, or otherwise, without the prior written permission of the AHIMA, 233 North Michigan Avenue, 21st Floor, Chicago, Illinois, 60601-5809 (https://secure.ahima.org/publications/reprint/index.aspx).

ISBN: 978-1-58426-771-3

AHIMA Product No.: AC400420

AHIMA Staff:
Jessica Block, MA, Production Development Editor
Megan Grennan, Managing Editor
James Pinnick, Vice President, Content and Product Development
Rachel Schratz, MA, Assistant Editor

Cover image: ©Volha Ramanchuk; iStock

Limit of Liability/Disclaimer of Warranty: This book is sold, as is, without warranty of any kind, either express or implied. While every precaution has been taken in the preparation of this book, the publisher and author assume no responsibility for errors or omissions. Neither is any liability assumed for damages resulting from the use of the information or instructions contained herein. It is further stated that the publisher and author are not responsible for any damage or loss to your data or your equipment that results directly or indirectly from your use of this book.

The websites listed in this book were current and valid as of the date of publication. However, webpage addresses and the information on them may change at any time. The user is encouraged to perform his or her own general web searches to locate any site addresses listed here that are no longer valid.

CPT® is a registered trademark of the American Medical Association. CCS® is a registered trademark of the American Health Information Management Association. All other copyrights and trademarks mentioned in this book are the possession of their respective owners. AHIMA makes no claim of ownership by mentioning products that contain such marks.

AHIMA certifications are administered by the AHIMA Commission on Certification for Health Informatics and Information Management (CCHIIM). The CCHIIM does not contribute to, review, or endorse any review books, review sessions, study guides, or other exam preparatory activities. Use of this product for AHIMA certification exam preparation in no way guarantees an exam candidate will earn a passing score on the examination.

For more information, including updates, about AHIMA Press publications, visit http://www.ahima.org/education/press.

American Health Information Management Association
233 North Michigan Avenue, 21st Floor
Chicago, Illinois 60601-5809
ahima.org

Contents

About the Contributing Editor iv
Acknowledgments..v
About the CCS Exam vi
How to Use This Book and Online Assessments viii

Introduction
    Steps for Success..1
    Make Plans for CCS Success 1
    Self-Evaluation Notes 2
    Coding Challenges 2
    A Note on *CCS Exam Preparation* Case Studies..3
    Medical Scenario Instructions for the CCS Certification Exam 3

Practice Questions
    Multiple-Choice Questions 6
    Case Studies 30

Exam 1
    Multiple-Choice Questions 68
    Case Studies 90

Exam 2
    Multiple-Choice Questions 140
    Case Studies 164

Answer Key
Practice
    Multiple-Choice Questions 206
    Case Studies 214
Exam 1
    Multiple-Choice Questions 217
    Case Studies 226
Exam 2
    Multiple-Choice Questions 230
    Case Studies 238

References 243

Online Assessments
    Practice Multiple-Choice Questions, Case Studies, and Answers
    Exam 1 Multiple-Choice Question, Case Studies, and Answers
    Exam 2 Multiple-Choice Questions, Case Studies, and Answers

About the Contributing Editor

Dianna M. Foley, RHIA, CCS, CDIP, CHPS has been an HIM professional for 20 years, holding jobs as coder, department supervisor, department director, and now as a coding consultant. She earned her bachelor's degree from the University of Cincinnati and subsequently achieved her RHIA, CHPS, CCS, and CDIP certifications. Ms. Foley previously served as the program director for medical coding and HIT at Eastern Gateway Community College. She is an AHIMA-approved ICD-10-CM/PCS trainer and is the coding education coordinator for OHIMA. Along with authoring this textbook, Ms. Foley authored *Health Information Management Case Studies,* Second Edition; coauthored *Basic ICD-10-CM and ICD-10-PCS Coding Exercises*, Sixth Edition; and was a technical editor for the 2017 edition of the *Clinical Coding Workout* book. In addition, Ms. Foley was a contributor to AHIMA's Code Update Rapid Design Project in 2016 and 2017, and as a member of AHIMA's Coding Roundtable Coordinators, she participated in updating the Coding Roundtable Coordinator's Toolkit in 2016 and 2018. Ms. Foley has also served on AHIMA's item writing, exam development, and standard setting committees. She has presented webinars for AHIMA and OHIMA on a variety of coding topics. She serves on the OHIMA board in capacities such as newsletter contributor, participant on the scholarship and awards committee, and facilitator of coding roundtables. Ms. Foley mentors new AHIMA members and provides monthly educational lectures to coders and clinical documentation specialists.

Acknowledgments

AHIMA Press wishes to thank the following individuals for being editors, reviewers, and publishers of previous editions of the *CCS Exam Success Review Book* and *CCS Exam Preparation*:

Jennifer Hornung Garvin, PhD, MBA, RHIA, CCS, CPHQ, CTR, FAHIMA
Shawn Wells, RHIT, CHDA
Elizabeth Forrestal, PhD, RHIA, CCS, FAHIMA
Kathy Arner, MCS, LPN, RHIT, CCS, CPC, CPMA
Genevive Badroe, CCA
Christine Staropoli, MS, RHIA, CCS
Angela Picard Carney, PhD, RHIA
Stephen Weiner, DO
Julian Wade Farrior, PhD
Pam Farrior, RPh
Aileen Stanton, CHCO, CCS, CCP
Pauline Graham, RHIT, CHCO, CCS, CCP
Becky Thorson, RHIT, CCS
Linda Donahue, RHIT, CCS, CCS-P, CPC
Christina Benjamin, MA, RHIA, CCS, CCS-P
Dasantila Sherifi, MBA, RHIA
Kay B. Leonard, RHIA
Anita Kang, RHIT
Patrice Jackson, RHIA, CHP, CCS, CHTS-TR, CHTS-PW, CHTS-IM, CMRS, CHAM
Kathryn A. DeVault, MSL, RHIA, CCS, CCS-P, PCS, FAHIMA
Melanie A. Endicott, MBA/HCM, RHIA, CCS, CCS-P, CDIP, CHDA, FAHIMA
Kelli Horn, RHIT, CCS
Dawn Moser, RHIA, CCS, CCS-P, CMRS
Maria Ward, MeD, RHIT, CCS-P
Lorraine Papazian-Boyce, MS, CPC
Dana Carcamo, RHIA, CCS
Tina Cressman, MALS, CCS, CCS-P, CPC, COC, CPC-P, CEMC, CPMA, CPEDC, CPC-I, MCS-P, MCS-I, CHEP

AHIMA Press would like to acknowledge and thank Suzanne Forrest, RHIA, CCS, CCS-P, CPC; Cari Greenwood, RHIA, CCS; Gretchen Jopp, MS, RHIA, CCS, CPC; and Mary Stanfill, MBI, RHIA, CCS, CCS-P, FAHIMA for their technical review of this edition.

About the CCS Exam

Coding professionals who pass the certified coding specialist (CCS) exam are professionals skilled in classifying medical data from patient records, generally in the hospital setting. These coding practitioners review patients' records and assign numeric codes for each diagnosis and procedure. To perform this task, they must possess expertise in the ICD-10-CM, ICD-10-PCS, and CPT coding systems. In addition, the CCS is knowledgeable of medical terminology, disease processes, and pharmacology. Hospitals or medical providers report coded data to insurance companies, or to the government in the case of Medicare and Medicaid recipients, for reimbursement of expenses. Researchers and public health officials also use coded medical data to monitor patterns and explore new interventions. Coding accuracy is thus highly important to healthcare organizations because of its impact on revenues and describing health outcomes, and certification is becoming an implicit industry standard. Accordingly, the CCS credential demonstrates tested data quality and integrity skills in a coding practitioner. The CCS certification exam assesses mastery proficiency in coding rather than entry-level skills. Professionals experienced in coding inpatient and outpatient records should consider obtaining this certification. For exam eligibility requirements, visit http://ahima.org/certification/CCS.

The National Commission for Certifying Agencies (NCCA) has granted accreditation to AHIMA's certified coding specialist (CCS) certification program for demonstrating compliance with the NCCA Standards for the Accreditation of Certification Programs. NCCA is the accrediting body of the Institute for Credentialing Excellence (formerly the National Organization for Competency Assurance).

The NCCA Standards were created in 1977 and updated in 2014 to ensure that certification programs adhere to modern standards of practice for the certification industry. AHIMA joins an elite group of more than 100 organizations representing more than 200 programs that have received and maintained NCCA accreditation. More information on the NCCA is available online at http://www.credentialingexcellence.org/ncca.

The Commission on Certification for Health Informatics and Information Management (CCHIIM) manages and sets the strategic direction for the certifications.

Certified Coding Specialist (CCS) Examination Content Outline

Number of Questions on exam:
- 97 multiple-choice questions (79 scored/18 pretest)
- 8 medical scenarios (6 scored/2 pretest)

Exam Time: 4 hours (no breaks)

Domain 1—Coding Knowledge and Skills (51.9%)

Tasks:

1. Apply diagnosis and procedure codes based on provider's documentation in the health record
2. Determine principal/primary diagnosis and procedure
3. Apply coding conventions/guidelines and regulatory guidance
4. Apply CPT/HCPCS modifiers to outpatient procedures
5. Sequence diagnoses and procedures

6. Apply present on admission (POA) guidelines
7. Address coding edits
8. Assign reimbursement classifications
9. Abstract pertinent data from health record
10. Recognize major conditions and co-morbidity (MCC) and conditions and co-morbidity (CC)

Domain 2—Coding Documentation (10.1%)

Tasks:

1. Review health record to assign diagnosis and procedure codes for an encounter
2. Review and address health record discrepancies

Domain 3—Provider Queries (8.9%)

Tasks:

1. Determine if a provider query is compliant
2. Analyze current documentation to identify query opportunities

Domain 4—Regulatory Compliance (29.1%)

Tasks:

1. Ensure integrity of health records
2. Apply payer-specific guidelines
3. Recognize patient safety indicators (PSIs) and hospital-acquired conditions (HACs) based on documentation
4. Ensure compliance with HIPAA guidelines
5. Ensure adherence to AHIMA's Standards of Ethical Coding
6. Apply the Uniform Hospital Discharge Data Set (UHDDS)

Medical Scenarios

1. Inpatient (33.33%)
2. Outpatient (33.33%)
3. Emergency Department (33.33%)

Books to Bring

For a full list of allowable code books, please see AHIMA's Certification website at http://www.ahima.org/certification/CCS.

Candidates without the required code books will not be permitted to test and will forfeit their application fees. Candidates who do not bring all the required books, or whose books do not have the correct year will not be allowed to test. For the most up-to-date exam information, visit http://www.ahima.org/certification/CCS.

How to Use This Book and Online Assessments

The CCS practice questions and practice exams in this book test knowledge of content pertaining to the CCS competencies published by AHIMA and available at ahima.org/certification. The multiple-choice practice questions and practice medical cases along with two practice exams are presented in a similar format to what might be found on the CCS exam.

This book contains a practice section and two complete practice exams, each comprised of 97 multiple-choice questions and 8 medical scenarios. Each multiple-choice question is identified with one of the four CCS domains, so you will be able to determine whether you need knowledge or skill building in particular areas of the exam domains. All answers include rationales and references for further guidance. Pursuing these references will help you build your knowledge and skills in specific domains.

To most effectively use this book, work through all of the practice questions first. This will help you identify areas in which you may need further preparation. For the questions that you answer incorrectly, read the associated references to help refresh your knowledge. After going through the practice questions, take one of the practice exams. Again, for the questions that you answer incorrectly, refresh your knowledge by reading the associated references and study resources.

The online assessments contain the same multiple-choice questions from the book. The practice questions and practice exams can be presented in random order, or you may choose to go through the questions in sequential order by domain. You may also choose to practice or test your skills on specific domains. For example, if you would like to build your skills in domain 2, you may choose only that domain's questions for a given practice session.

Introduction

The purpose of this book is to provide practice exercises for the certified coding specialist (CCS) exam through a review of important ICD-10-CM, ICD-10-PCS, and CPT coding material. Two simulations of the CCS exam are included in this book to help you improve test performance within the context of the four-hour exam. The content of this book is not intended to predict what will be on the CCS exam, and utilizing *CCS Exam Preparation* does not guarantee a passing score. However, *CCS Exam Preparation* does provide a focused method of preparing for the exam through review, practice, and exam simulation.

Steps for Success

1. Review basic coding principles in coding books and then test yourself via the exercises provided in this book and online assessments.
2. Review relevant American Hospital Association *Coding Clinic for ICD-10-CM and ICD-10-PCS* articles. Read as many issues of the *Coding Clinic* as possible, but be sure to start with the most recent issue and work backward. As noted, the *Coding Clinic* articles used to develop the 2020 CCS exam end with the fourth quarter of 2019.
3. Review the *ICD-10-CM Official Guidelines for Coding and Reporting*, which can be found at https://www.cms.gov/Medicare/Coding/ICD10/Downloads/2020-ICD10-Coding-Guidelines-.pdf as well as the *ICD-10-PCS Official Guidelines for Coding and Reporting*, which can be found at https://www.cms.gov/Medicare/Coding/ICD10/2020-ICD-10-PCS.html. The national standards for coding practice are provided in *Coding Clinic for ICD-10-CM and ICD-10-PCS* and the *Official Coding Guidelines*. These resources establish the correct answers related to ICD-10-CM and ICD-10-PCS on the CCS exam.
4. Review an educational text on CPT and complete exercises for areas in which more skill is needed. Review the guidelines section of each section of the CPT code book to ensure adequate knowledge of the details of each area.
5. Review the American Medical Association *CPT Assistant* from the most recent issue going backward as far as possible.
6. Complete the introductory exercises and practice questions in this book.
7. To prepare psychologically for the experience of taking the four-hour CCS exam, simulate the experience by completing a practice exam *in one sitting*. Along with practice questions and case studies, this book contains two practice exams (each with 97 multiple-choice questions and 8 medical scenarios). The online assessment contains the two complete exams and practice questions that can be presented in sequential order (by domain) or random order.
8. Follow up with the references and other CCS study resources. Ask AHIMA-approved ICD-10-CM/PCS trainers and CCS-credentialed professionals for clarification on items that are unclear.

For more information on the exam, refer to the About the CCS Exam section earlier in this book or visit http://ahima.org/certification/CCS. Another valuable resource is the AHIMA Engage Communities for CCS Exam Preparation.

Make Plans for CCS Success

In order to develop a good plan of study, it is important to reflect on what you have read so far. Use a calendar to determine how much time you have to prepare.

- How many hours can you spend per week studying?
- How many weeks do you have to study before the exam? (Exclude weeks when you have personal or family events.)

Good preparation using the steps for success can help you achieve a successful exam experience!

Introduction

Self-Evaluation Notes

Each person who studies for the CCS exam has a different skill set. One of the goals for using this book is to determine your areas of weakness. Strategies can then be developed to make weak areas stronger. Take a few minutes to complete this self-evaluation so that your specific needs can be addressed. Use this self-evaluation to help gather resources before working through the remainder of this book.

I need more practice in these areas:

1.
2.
3.

I can strengthen these areas by:

1.
2.
3.

I need these resources to help me:

1.
2.
3.

You may find it beneficial to reassess your strengths and weaknesses after each exam. That way, you can track the improvements that you are making and reidentify potential problem areas.

Coding Challenges

The following is an overview of some potentially challenging coding issues. When possible, obtain the reference materials listed in the back of this book and utilize them. Creating a study schedule and reviewing materials that address your weaknesses will enable you to achieve your goals.

In order to do well on the multiple-choice section of this book, reference material related to the exam content should be memorized. It is not possible to memorize everything, so developing a study strategy is important. Be sure to read the About the CCS Exam section earlier in this book to fully understand the exam contents and what should be coded in the medical cases. Determine weak areas and study to improve those areas. Focus on clinical scenarios and reimbursement topics that would apply to the "average" hospital.

Code books are allowed during the CCS exam. Refer to the AHIMA Certification website (http://www.ahima.org/certification) for a current list of allowable code books. Furthermore, materials in code books must be permanently affixed inside your code books. Remember, too, that you will need to gain speed using the code books because an encoder is not used to assign codes during the exam. In order to hone this skill, practice coding exercises by timing yourself to evaluate your speed and accuracy using actual code books.

The following are highlights to remember:

- Knowledge of MS-DRGs and APCs are important. Which MS-DRGs will be affected by major comorbidities or complications (MCCs) and complications or comorbidities (CCs) is key information. You should have a general idea about common MS-DRGs for the average hospital in the United States and the reimbursement methodology of APCs. For example, what status indicators mean and how to assign evaluation and management (E/M) levels if given a template.
- Generally, cases on the exam reflect common cases that a coder in an average hospital would code. Determine if you have a knowledge deficit in any common coding areas because your facility does not treat that type of patient. For example, some facilities do not provide services for newborns, deliveries, heart catheterizations, coronary artery bypass grafts (CABGs), or neonatal intensive care. If you work in such a facility, you will need to strategize how to gather expertise in these areas. One way to gain expertise is to review the coding exercises in a basic coding book and to use an encoder to determine the MS-DRGs associated with the exercises.

Introduction

Outpatient Prospective Payment System

The outpatient prospective payment system (OPPS), for ambulatory care, began to be used for Medicare in August 2000. This system uses the ambulatory payment classifications (APCs) for reimbursement for hospital-based outpatient services such as outpatient surgery, emergency department visits, outpatient clinic visits, and outpatient ancillary tests. Some highlights of this system are listed here:

- APCs are similar to MS-DRGs in that they are both prospective payment methodologies and both have relative weights.
- APCs are different from MS-DRGs because outpatients can have multiple APCs for a given encounter, whereas an inpatient can have only one MS-DRG.
- APCs are generated for many services, such as x-rays, medical tests, clinic or emergency visits, surgical procedures, devices, drugs and biologicals, and partial hospitalizations.
- The billing number is the connecting identifier for a given patient's encounter that results in multiple APCs.

Status indicators reimbursed by the OPPS denote what type of service was provided and assist in determining the payment. Status indicators include, among others: X, ancillary; V, clinic or emergency department visit; T, significant procedure that is discounted when other T procedures are provided (the first procedure is paid at a rate of 100 percent whereas the second and those thereafter are paid at 50 percent); S, significant procedure that is paid at 100 percent and is not discounted; P, partial hospitalization; H, Pass-through device categories; G, drugs/biologicals; K, Non-pass-through drugs and non-implantable biological, including therapeutic radiopharmaceuticals. Please visit the CMS web page (noted in the References in this book) for more information and a complete list of status indicators.

A Note on *CCS Exam Preparation* Case Studies

Eight medical scenarios are a component of both the book and the certification exam. Three categories of cases are presented for coding: inpatient, outpatient, and emergency department scenarios. The answers are grouped into three categories: principal or first-listed diagnosis, secondary or additional diagnosis codes, and procedure codes. The sequencing of codes within the categories is not tested on the actual certification exam or on the online assessment that accompanies this book. *CCS Exam Preparation* also includes guidelines for coding the case studies, listed below, that are not included on the 2020 CCS exam.

The *CCS Exam Preparation* book contains two full exams and a practice exam with eight case studies each. The documentation-based cases are one of the most valuable aspects of the materials presented in the book and corresponding online assessment.

The medical scenario instructions for the CCS exam launching in May 2020 are reprinted here for review, and other exam preparation materials, including the list of allowable code books, can be found at http://www.ahima.org/certification/CCS.

Instructions and official guidelines for coding health records are included in the following resources: ICD-10-CM and ICD-10-PCS, CPT, UHDDS, *Coding Clinic*, and *CPT Assistant*.

However, hospitals and other organizations may develop their own procedures in the absence of approved guidelines.

Medical Scenario Instructions for the CCS Certification Exam

Read the clinical scenario. Many of the cases will be longer than the screen. Please make sure to scroll all the way to the bottom of the cases to read all of the information. Following the clinical scenario are two to three questions. The questions will ask you to code the:

Principal or first-listed diagnosis: Select only one diagnosis for this question. All cases will ask you this question.

Additional diagnosis codes: Select as many as are appropriate. You may select "none" if no additional diagnosis codes apply to the case. Over-coding will result in a loss of points. Some cases may exclude this question, but please note that "none" is almost always an option for this question.

Introduction

Procedure codes: Select as many as are appropriate. You may select "none" if no procedure codes apply to the case. Over-coding will result in a loss of points. Some cases may exclude this question, but please note that "none" is almost always an option for this question.

The sequencing of codes is not being tested in this section. Please only select the appropriate codes. No points will be awarded for over- or under-coding.

Please note that the number of options available to select the codes from is not an indicator of the number of correct options and that in some instances "none" should be selected as the correct answer.

For this edition we included only those procedure codes that have been specified in past years as noted below.

Guidelines for Coding the *CCS Exam Preparation* Case Studies

For inpatient cases:

- Code all procedures that fall within the code range 001 through 10Y.
- Do not code procedures that fall within the code range 2W0 (Placement) through HZ9 (Substance Abuse Treatment). Do code procedures in the following ranges:
    - Cholangiograms
    - Retrogrades, urinary systems
    - Arteriography and angiography
    - Radiation therapy
    - Psychiatric therapy
    - Alcohol/drug detoxification and rehabilitation
    - Insertion of endotracheal tube
    - Other lavage of bronchus and trachea
    - Mechanical ventilation
    - ESWL
    - Chemotherapy

For ambulatory care cases:

- Do not assign ICD-10-PCS procedure codes.
- Assign CPT codes for all surgical procedures that fall in the surgery section.
- Assign CPT codes from the following *only if* indicated on the case cover sheet:
    - Anesthesia section
    - Medicine section
    - Evaluation and management services section
    - Radiology section
    - Laboratory and pathology section
- Assign CPT/HCPCS modifiers for hospital-based facilities, if applicable (regardless of payer).
- Do not assign HCPCS Level II (alphanumeric) codes.

CCS

PRACTICE QUESTIONS

Practice Questions

A blank answer sheet for these multiple-choice questions can be found on page 27.

Domain 1 — Coding Knowledge and Skills

1. A 12-year-old boy was seen in an ambulatory surgical center for pain in his right arm. The x-ray showed fracture of ulna. Patient underwent closed reduction of fracture right proximal ulna and an elbow-to-finger cast was applied. What diagnostic and procedure codes should be assigned?

S52.101A	Unspecified fracture of upper end of right radius, initial encounter for closed fracture
S52.101B	Unspecified fracture of upper end of right radius, initial encounter for open fracture
S52.001A	Unspecified fracture of upper end of right ulna, initial encounter for closed fracture
S52.001B	Unspecified fracture of upper end of right ulna, initial encounter for open fracture
0PSH0ZZ	Reposition right radius, open approach
0PSK0ZZ	Reposition right ulna, open approach
24670	Closed treatment of ulnar fracture, proximal end (eg, olecranon or coronoid process(es)); without manipulation
24675	Closed treatment of ulnar fracture, proximal end (eg, olecranon or coronoid process(es)); with manipulation
25560	Closed treatment of radial and ulnar shaft fractures; without manipulation
29075	Application, cast; elbow to finger (short arm)

   a. S52.101A, S52.001A, 0PSK0ZZ
   b. S52.101B, S52.001B, 0PSH0ZZ
   c. S52.101B, S52.001B, 25560, 29075
   d. S52.001A, 24675

2. A 75-year-old male patient was admitted from a nursing home with dehydration and dysphagia due to a previous stroke. During hospitalization, the patient was rehydrated and transferred back to the nursing home. What codes should be assigned?

   a. E86.0, I69.390, R13.19
   b. E86.1, I69.391, R13.10
   c. E86.9, I69.390, R13.19
   d. E86.0, I69.391, R13.10

3. Sepsis due to the presence of an indwelling urinary catheter with a positive blood culture reflected in the progress notes as *Staphylococcus aureus* sepsis. What codes should be assigned?

   a. T83.511A, A41.01
   b. T83.511A, A41.9
   c. T83.510A, R78.81
   d. T81.4XXA, A41.01

4. A laparoscopic tubal ligation is completed. What is the correct CPT code assignment?

49320	Laparoscopy, abdomen, peritoneum, and omentum, diagnostic, with or without collection of specimen(s) by brushing or washing (separate procedure)
58662	Laparoscopy, surgical; with fulguration or excision of lesions of the ovary, pelvic viscera, or peritoneal surface by any method
58670	Laparoscopy, surgical; with fulguration of oviducts (with or without transection)
58671	Laparoscopy, surgical; with occlusion of oviducts by device (eg, band, clip, or Falope ring)

   a. 49320, 58662
   b. 58670
   c. 58671
   d. 49320

5. A patient is admitted to an acute-care facility with chest pain. The patient was awakened from sleep by the pain. This was the patient's first experience with chest pain. The patient was given two nitroglycerin tablets in the emergency department. The chest pain was not relieved, resulting in the diagnosis of new onset unstable angina. Serial creatine phosphokinase was normal. Following a left cardiac catheterization with fluoroscopic angiogram of multiple coronary arteries with low osmolar contrast, the patient is found to have arteriosclerotic coronary artery disease. What ICD-10-CM and PCS codes should be assigned?

   a. I25.10, 4A023N7, B2111ZZ
   b. I25.110, 4A023N7, B211Y10
   c. I25.110, 4A023N7, B2111ZZ
   d. I25.110, 4A023N6, B2111ZZ

6. Normal twin delivery at 30 weeks. Both babies were delivered vaginally and were liveborn. What conditions should have codes assigned?

O30.003	Twin pregnancy, unspecified number of placenta and unspecified number of amniotic sacs, third trimester
O30.009	Twin pregnancy, unspecified number of placenta and unspecified number of amniotic sacs, unspecified trimester
O60.14X0	Preterm labor third trimester with preterm delivery third trimester, not applicable or unspecified
O60.14X1	Preterm labor third trimester with preterm delivery third trimester, fetus 1
O60.14X2	Preterm labor third trimester with preterm delivery third trimester, fetus 2
O80	Encounter for full-term uncomplicated delivery
Z3A.30	30 weeks gestation of pregnancy
Z37.0	Single live birth
Z37.2	Twins, both liveborn

   a. O80, Z3A.30, Z37.0
   b. O30.003, O60.14X0, Z3A.30, Z37.2
   c. O60.14X1, O60.14X2 O30.003, Z3A.30, Z37.2
   d. O80, O30.009, Z3A.30, Z37.2

Practice Questions

7. A patient is admitted with metastatic carcinoma from breast to liver with previous bilateral mastectomy and no reoccurrence at the primary site. In the progress note of day three, the physician indicates that patient now has pneumonia and begins treatment with an antibiotic which will be continued on discharge. What is the proper coding and sequencing of this admission?

    a. C78.6, Z85.3, Z90.13
    b. C78.7, J18.9, Z85.3, Z90.13
    c. J18.9, C78.7, Z90.13
    d. C78.7, Z85.3, Z90.10

8. Patient admitted with syncope due to taking Valium in combination with an over-the-counter antihistamine, taken as directed on the package but without consulting a healthcare provider. What are the correct codes and sequencing for this admission?

    a. R55, T42.4X1A, T45.0X1A
    b. T42.4X1A, T45.0X1A, R55
    c. T45.0X1A, T42.4X1A
    d. R55, T42.4X6A, T45.0X5A

9. 50-year-old woman with a diagnosis of metastatic ovarian cancer to the pleura has an outpatient thoracoscopic pleurodesis performed. What is the correct coding and sequencing?

    a. C56.9, C78.2, 32650
    b. C78.2, C56.9, 32650
    c. C78.2, C56.9, 32661
    d. C56.9, C78.2, 32609

10. A patient with acute respiratory failure, hypertension, and congestive heart failure is admitted for intubation and ventilation. The patient's heart failure is stable on current medications. What are the correct diagnosis codes and sequencing?

Code	Description
I10	Essential hypertension
I11.0	Hypertensive heart with heart failure
I50.9	Heart failure, unspecified
J96.00	Acute respiratory failure, unspecified whether with hypoxia or hypercapnia
J96.20	Acute and chronic respiratory failure, unspecified whether with hypoxia or hypercapnia

    a. J96.00, I11.0, I50.9
    b. I50.9, J96.00, I10
    c. J96.20, I10, I50.9
    d. I50.9, J96.20, I11.0

11. A 34-year-old woman delivered a live-born, term baby boy (39 weeks) with macrosomia. She had a hemorrhage following a low forceps delivery with episiotomy but prior to expulsion of the placenta. What are the appropriate codes and sequencing for this record?

    a. O67.8, O36.63X0, Z37.0, 10D07Z3, 0W8NXZZ
    b. Z37.0, O67.9, O36.63X1, Z3A.39, 10D07Z3, 0W8NXZZ
    c. O36.80X0, O67.9, Z37.0, Z3A.39, 0W8NXZZ, 10D07Z3
    d. O67.9, O36.63X0, Z37.0, Z3A.39, 10D07Z3, 0W8NXZZ

12. A 64-year-old female was discharged with the final diagnosis of acute renal failure and hypertension. What coding guideline applies?

    a. Use combination code of hypertension and chronic renal failure.

    b. Use separate codes for hypertension and chronic renal failure.

    c. Use separate codes for hypertension and acute renal failure.

    d. Use combination code for hypertension and acute renal failure.

13. A patient was discharged from the same-day-surgery unit with the following diagnoses: posterior subcapsular, mature, incipient, senile cataract right eye, diabetes mellitus, hypertension, and was treated for mild acute renal failure. Which codes are correct?

Code	Description
E11.36	Type 2 diabetes mellitus with diabetic cataract
E11.29	Type 2 diabetes mellitus with other diabetic kidney complication
E11.9	Type 2 diabetes mellitus without complications
H25.9	Unspecified age-related cataract
H25.21	Age-related cataract, morgagnian type, right eye
H25.041	Posterior subcapsular polar age-related cataract, right eye
I10	Essential hypertension
I12.9	Hypertensive chronic kidney disease with stage 1 through stage 4, or unspecified chronic kidney disease
N17.9	Acute kidney failure, unspecified

    a. H25.21, E11.29, I12.9, N17.9

    b. E11.36, H25.041, I10, N17.9

    c. H25.9, E11.29, I12.9, N17.9

    d. H25.041, E11.9, I12.9

14. Current Procedural Terminology (CPT) defines a separate procedure as which of the following?

    a. Procedure considered an integral part of a more major service

    b. Provision of anesthesia

    c. Procedure that requires an add-on code

    d. A surgical procedure performed in conjunction with an E&M visit

15. Documentation from the nursing or other allied health professionals' notes can be used to provide specificity for code assignment for which of the following diagnoses?

    a. Body mass index (BMI)

    b. Malnutrition

    c. Aspiration pneumonia

    d. Fatigue

16. A 30-year-old patient was seen in the emergency department for recurrent seizures. The patient also had tic douloureux. What codes should be assigned?

    a. R56.9, G50.0

    b. G40.909, G50.0

    c. R56.9, G50.8

    d. G40.919, F95.9

Practice Questions

17. A laparoscopic cholecystectomy was performed. What is the correct ICD-10-PCS code?

    > 0FB40ZZ   Excision of gallbladder, open approach
    > 0FB44ZZ   Excision of gallbladder, percutaneous endoscopic approach
    > 0FT40ZZ   Resection of gallbladder, open approach
    > 0FT44ZZ   Resection of gallbladder, percutaneous endoscopic approach

    a. 0FB40ZZ

    b. 0FT40ZZ

    c. 0FT44ZZ

    d. 0FB44ZZ

18. A 59-year-old man who works in construction is diagnosed with basal cell carcinoma of the eye. An excision of basal cell carcinoma of the left upper eyelid was performed with an excised diameter of 1.9 cm and single layer closure. What codes and modifiers should be assigned?

    a. C44.121, 11622-E2

    b. C44.1191, 11642-E1

    c. C44.1191, 11640-E1

    d. C44.121, 11642-E2

19. Carcinoma of multiple overlapping sites of the bladder. Diagnostic cystoscopy and transurethral fulguration of bladder lesions over the dome and posterior wall (1.9 cm) was completed. A biopsy was taken of a lesion in the lateral wall. What modifier should be added to the biopsy procedure code?

    a. −50, Bilateral procedure

    b. −51, Multiple procedures

    c. −59, Distinct procedural service

    d. −99, Multiple modifiers

20. A bronchoscopy with multiple biopsies of the left bronchus was completed and revealed adenocarcinoma. What, if any, modifier should be added to the procedure code billed by the facility?

    a. −59, Distinct procedural service

    b. −51, Multiple procedures

    c. −76, Repeat procedure or service by same physician

    d. No modifiers should be reported

21. A patient is admitted with fever and urinary burning. Urosepsis is suspected. The discharge diagnosis is *Escherichia coli*, urinary tract infection; sepsis ruled out. Which of the following represents the diagnoses to report for this encounter and the appropriate sequencing of the codes for those conditions?

    a. Fever, urinary burning, urosepsis
    b. Fever, urinary burning, sepsis
    c. *Escherichia coli* sepsis
    d. Urinary tract infection, *Escherichia coli*

22. A patient was admitted to the emergency department for abdominal pain with diarrhea and was diagnosed with infectious gastroenteritis. In addition to gastroenteritis, the final diagnostic statement included angina and chronic obstructive pulmonary disease. List the diagnoses that would be coded and their correct sequence.

    a. Abdominal pain, infectious gastroenteritis, chronic obstructive pulmonary disease, angina
    b. Infectious gastroenteritis, chronic obstructive pulmonary disease, angina
    c. Gastroenteritis, abdominal pain, angina
    d. Diarrhea, chronic obstructive pulmonary disease, angina

23. A patient was admitted to the endoscopy unit for a screening colonoscopy. During the colonoscopy, polyps of the colon were found and a polypectomy was performed. What diagnostic codes should be used and how should they be sequenced?

Z12.11	Encounter for screening for malignant neoplasm of colon
D12.6	Benign neoplasm of colon, unspecified
Z86.010	Personal history of colonic polyps

    a. Z12.11, Z86.010
    b. D12.6, Z12.11, Z86.010
    c. Z12.11, D12.6
    d. D12.6, Z12.11

24. A 30-year-old patient with acquired immunodeficiency syndrome (AIDS), asymptomatic at this time, is admitted for repair of inguinal hernia. The procedure performed was a right indirect inguinal herniorrhaphy via open approach. What are the correct codes and sequencing for this scenario?

    a. B20, K40.90, 0YQ5XZZ
    b. K40.90, B20, 0YQ50ZZ
    c. Z21, K40.90, 0YQ5XZZ
    d. K40.90, Z21, 0YQ50ZZ

Practice Questions

25. The patient is admitted for chest pain and is found to have an acute inferior myocardial infarction with coronary artery disease and atrial fibrillation. After the atrial fibrillation was controlled and the patient was stabilized, the patient underwent a CABG ×2 from aorta to the right anterior descending and right obtuse, using the left greater saphenous vein which was harvested via an open approach. Cardiopulmonary bypass was utilized. The appropriate sequencing and ICD codes for the hospitalization would be:

Code	Description
I25.10	Atherosclerotic heart disease of native coronary artery without angina pectoris
I21.19	ST elevation (STEMI) myocardial infarction involving other coronary artery of inferior wall
I22.1	Subsequent ST elevation (STEMI) myocardial infarction of inferior wall
I21.3	ST elevation (STEMI) myocardial infarction, of unspecified site
I22.9	Subsequent ST elevation (STEMI) myocardial infarction of unspecified site
I48.91	Unspecified atrial fibrillation
R07.9	Chest pain, unspecified
02100AW	Bypass coronary artery, one artery from aorta with autologous arterial tissue, open approach
021109W	Bypass coronary artery, two arteries from aorta with autologous venous tissue, open approach
06BQ0ZZ	Excision of left saphenous vein, open approach
5A1221Z	Performance of cardiac output, continuous

    a. R07.9, I21.3, I48.91, I22.9, 02100AW, 5A1221Z

    b. I21.19, I48.91, I22.9, 02100AW

    c. I21.19, I25.10, I48.91, 021109W, 06BQ0ZZ, 5A1221Z

    d. I22.1, I48.91, I21.19, 021109W

26. Twin newborns are born prematurely at 32 weeks via cesarean section. 1,002g was the birth weight of the first twin, whose mate was stillborn. The baby was admitted to the nursery from the delivery room. The baby was also treated for jaundice due to ABO incompatibility. What codes should be assigned and what is the proper sequencing?

    a. Z38.31, P07.14, P07.35, P55.1

    b. Z38.01, P07.35, P07.14, P55.8

    c. P05.04, P07.35, Z38.31, P55.1

    d. Z38.31, P07.14, P07.33, P55.1

27. A patient is admitted with hemoptysis. A bronchoscopy with transbronchial biopsy of the lower lobe was undertaken that revealed squamous cell carcinoma of the right lung. Which conditions should be identified as present on admission?

Code	Description
C34.30	Malignant neoplasm of lower lobe, unspecified bronchus or lung
C34.31	Malignant neoplasm of lower lobe, right bronchus or lung
P26.9	Unspecified pulmonary hemorrhage originating in the perinatal period
R04.2	Hemoptysis

    a. C34.31, R04.2

    b. R04.2

    c. C34.31

    d. C34.30, P26.9, R04.2

28. A condition is considered present on admission when it is:

    a. The principal diagnosis
    b. In accordance with medical staff bylaws
    c. A condition that occurs prior to an inpatient admission
    d. Present within three days after admission

29. A newborn is diagnosed with meconium aspiration at birth. What is the appropriate POA indicator for the meconium aspiration?

    a. Y
    b. N
    c. U
    d. W

30. A woman is admitted to the hospital for an exacerbation of COPD and mentions a lump she has noticed in her right breast. While she in the hospital, a biopsy is done of the breast lump and a diagnosis of ductal carcinoma is made. What is the POA assignment for the carcinoma?

    a. Y
    b. N
    c. U
    d. W

31. The use of the outpatient code editor (OCE) is designed to:

    a. Correct documentation of home health visits
    b. Facilitate reporting of adverse drug events
    c. Reduce the use of computer assisted coding
    d. Identify incomplete or incorrect claims

32. Medicare's identification of medically necessary services is outlined in:

    a. Program transmittals
    b. Claims processing manual
    c. Local coverage determinations
    d. National Correct Coding Initiative

33. Medically unlikely edits are used to identify:

    a. Pairs of procedure codes that should not be billed together
    b. Maximum units of service for a HCPCS code
    c. Diagnoses that don't meet medical necessity
    d. Procedure and gender discrepancies

34. National Correct Coding Initiative (NCCI) Edits are released how often?

    a. Monthly
    b. Quarterly
    c. Semi-annually
    d. Annually

Practice Questions

35. In 2000, the Centers for Medicare and Medicaid Services (CMS) issued the final rule on the outpatient prospective payment system (OPPS). The final rule:

    a. Identified the payment structure for long-term care
    b. Divided outpatient services into fixed payment groups
    c. Created less opportunity for health information management professionals
    d. Facilitated greater use of ICD-9-CM procedure codes

36. Diagnostic-related groups (DRGs) and ambulatory patient classifications (APCs) are similar in that they are both:

    a. Determined by HCPCS codes
    b. Focused on hospital outpatients
    c. Focused on hospital inpatients
    d. Prospective payment systems

37. Medicare exerts control of provider reimbursement through adjustment of this component of the resource-based relative value scale (RBRVS).

    a. Conversion factor
    b. Geographic adjustment
    c. Relative value unit
    d. Practice expense

38. The process of collecting data elements from a source document is known as:

    a. Extracting
    b. Mining
    c. Abstracting
    d. Drilling

39. What piece of claims data from Hospital A alerts a payer that the patient was transferred to Hospital B?

    a. Admission source
    b. Admit diagnosis
    c. Discharge disposition
    d. Discharge diagnosis

Use the following table to answer questions 40 and 41.

Admission

Source Code	Admission Source Definition
1	Non-health care facility
2	Clinic
4	Transfer from Hospital
5	Transfer from Skilled or Intermediate Facility
6	Transfer from another Health Care Facility
7	Emergency Room
8	Court/Law Enforcement
E	Transfer from Ambulatory Surgery
F	Transfer from Hospice

40. What admission source code would be used when a patient is admitted to the facility from home?

    a. 1
    b. 2
    c. 6
    d. F

41. A terminally ill patient under hospice care is admitted to Hospital A for palliative care. What is the correct admission source code for the admission to Hospital A?

    a. 1
    b. 2
    c. 6
    d. F

42. When a patient is transferred from an acute-care facility to a skilled nursing facility, what abstracted data element can impact the DRG assignment?

    a. Admission source
    b. Patient's blood type
    c. Discharge disposition
    d. Patient's age

43. For a patient with a principal diagnosis of septicemia, reporting which of the following procedures will have the greatest impact on the MS-DRG?

    a. Excision of left main bronchus, percutaneous endoscopic approach, diagnostic (0BB74ZX)
    b. Excision of toe nail, external approach (0HBRXZZ)
    c. Extraction of perineum skin, external approach (0HD9XZZ)
    d. Respiratory ventilation, greater than 96 consecutive hours (5A1955Z)

44. Which of the following is considered a complication or comorbidity?

    a. Hypokalemia
    b. Dehydration
    c. Hypernatremia
    d. Fluid overload

Use the following scenario to answer questions 45 and 46.

A patient is admitted for a cerebral infarction. Residual effects at discharge include aphasia and dysphagia. The patient developed acute diastolic congestive heart failure while admitted and was treated with Lasix in addition to being given Betapace for his long-standing hypertension.

45. Which condition is considered a major complication comorbidity?

    a. Cerebral infarction
    b. Acute diastolic congestive heart failure
    c. Hypertension
    d. Dysphagia

Practice Questions

46. Which condition meets the definition of comorbidity?

    a. Cerebral infarction

    b. Acute diastolic congestive heart failure

    c. Hypertension

    d. Dysphagia

Domain 2 Coding Documentation

47. A patient was admitted from the emergency department because of chest pain. Following blood work, it was determined that the patient had elevated CK-MB enzymes. The EKG shows nonspecific ST changes. What type of diagnosis might this indicate?

    a. Unstable angina

    b. Myocardial infarction

    c. Congestive heart failure

    d. Mitral valve stenosis

48. A patient is admitted to the psychiatric unit of an acute-care facility. Almost every day for the past month, the patient has experienced loss of interest in most or all activities, which is a change from her prior level of functioning. She has also gained 15 lbs, has difficulty falling asleep, feels fatigued, and has difficulty making decisions. What potential diagnosis most closely fits the patient's overall symptoms?

    a. Insomnia

    b. Major depression

    c. Reye's syndrome

    d. Bipolar disorder

49. A patient is admitted to the hospital complaining of abdominal pain. Following evaluation, it was determined that the patient had an obstruction of the left colon due to adhesions from a prior abdominal surgery. The patient underwent laparotomy with lysis of adhesions. What conditions and procedures should be coded?

    a. Abdominal pain, abdominal adhesions, abdominal obstruction, laparotomy, lysis of adhesions

    b. Abdominal adhesions, abdominal obstruction, postoperative complications of the digestive system, laparotomy, lysis of adhesions

    c. Abdominal adhesions with obstruction, lysis of adhesions

    d. Abdominal adhesions, abdominal obstruction, postoperative complications of the digestive system, lysis of adhesions

Domain 2

50. A patient is diagnosed with infertility due to endometriosis and undergoes an outpatient laparoscopic laser destruction of pelvic endometriosis. In order to code this encounter accurately, what steps must the coder take?

    a. Review the operative report to determine what procedure codes to use. Determine the site or sites of endometriosis so codes with the highest specificity may be assigned. Use infertility as a principal diagnosis.

    b. Review the operative report to determine where the laser was used in the pelvis so the site or sites of endometriosis can be specified. Assign a principal diagnosis of infertility.

    c. Review the operative report to determine where the laser was used in the pelvis so the site or sites of endometriosis can be specified as principal. Assign a secondary diagnosis of infertility.

    d. Review the operative report to determine what procedure codes to use. Determine the site or sites of endometriosis so codes with the highest specificity may be assigned. Assign endometriosis as the principal diagnosis. Assign infertility as a secondary condition.

51. In order to accurately code a cardiac catheterization, in addition to the approach and the side of the heart into which the catheter was inserted, what else needs to be determined?

    a. The type of anesthesia used
    b. If additional procedures were performed
    c. The duration of the procedure
    d. Documentation that stents were considered

52. A female patient is admitted for a second-degree cystocele. A repair is performed. Which report provides the documentation necessary to accurately code the repair?

    a. History and physical
    b. Discharge summary
    c. Consultation
    d. Operative report

53. To accurately report wound closures with CPT codes, in addition to knowing the site and length of the closure, what other information is necessary?

    a. If anesthesia was used and what kind
    b. The repair type: simple, intermediate, or complex
    c. The supplies that were used
    d. If exploration of tendons or blood vessels occurred

54. A 64-year-old female is admitted to the hospital with nausea, vomiting, and edema. Lab values indicate the patient has dehydration. The patient takes Lisinopril as prescribed along with Levothyroxine for hypothyroidism. On the discharge summary, the final diagnoses of acute renal failure, hypothyroidism and dehydration are documented. What discrepancy should a coding professional note in this documentation?

    a. There is not enough detail in the documentation to assign the dehydration.
    b. There is no explanation for the patient's vomiting.
    c. There is no correlating diagnosis for the Lisinopril.
    d. The nausea, vomiting, and edema are indicative of chronic renal failure not acute.

Practice Questions

55. A patient comes in with right upper quadrant pain, nausea, and vomiting. An x-ray confirms inflammation in the gallbladder. The patient has been dealing with episodes like this for the past six months. The final diagnosis in the discharge statement is appendicitis. What discrepancy is noted in this record?

    a. The diagnosis indicates acute appendicitis
    b. There is no discrepancy, code the appendicitis
    c. The diagnosis indicates chronic appendicitis
    d. The diagnosis indicates acute on chronic cholecystitis

56. *Refer to question 55.* What should be done to correct the discrepancy?

    a. Since the patient came in with pain, it is appropriate to assign the code for acute appendicitis
    b. A query should be issued to determine the diagnosis as it seems appendicitis is incorrect
    c. A clinical documentation improvement specialist should be contacted to verify the diagnosis
    d. There is no discrepancy, code the appendicitis

57. A resident physician continually documents "CHF" without further clarification in patients' medical records. What is the most likely rationale for this documentation practice?

    a. No problem exists with this documentation as CHF without further clarification is acceptable.
    b. The resident is not qualified to make a more definitive determination of the type of CHF.
    c. The resident lacks knowledge regarding the need for further clarification.
    d. There is not enough information to determine the type of CHF.

58. A patient is scheduled for elective surgery for cataract removal of the left eye. The operative report indicates the surgery on the right eye is performed with the use of phacoemulsification and intraocular lens insertion. What discrepancy is noted in this documentation?

    a. The use of irrigation and aspiration is not mentioned
    b. No mention of implantation of intraocular lens
    c. No indication if general anesthesia was used
    d. Laterality is not in agreement

Domain 3 Provider Queries

59. An inpatient progress note on day two states there is a stage three pressure ulcer of the sacrum that requires debridement. The coding professional composes a query to determine if this condition was present on admission (POA) by asking the physician if the pressure ulcer listed in the progress note of day two was present on admission—yes or no? Is that an acceptable query? Why or why not?

    a. No. Yes/no queries are not acceptable in any circumstances.
    b. No. Yes/no queries require clinical indicators.
    c. Yes. Yes/no queries may be used to established POA status.
    d. Yes. Yes/no queries are the preferred query format for all queries.

60. Multiple choice queries must supply how many choices in order to be compliant?

    a. 3
    b. 4
    c. 5
    d. No specific number

61. Compliant queries include which of the following?

    a. Comparison of reimbursement amounts
    b. Relevant clinical indicators
    c. Potential impact on quality scores
    d. Impact on physician licensure

62. Examine the following query and determine if it is compliant and why:

    Dr. Reynolds, is it possible that this patient has acute, post-operative blood loss anemia based on the drop in hemoglobin and hematocrit that occurred after surgery as noted in the lab report? Yes or no?

    a. Yes, because the query provides clinical indicators for the additional diagnosis.
    b. Yes, because the physician has the option to choose yes or no.
    c. No, because the query is leading and inappropriately includes the term "possible" in the question.
    d. No, because yes and no queries are not acceptable.

63. Which of the following make a query compliant?

    a. Keeping the question vague so the physician has an opportunity to use his discretion when responding
    b. Explaining why the requested diagnosis is necessary to achieve a higher reimbursement
    c. Addressing the impact the query has on quality indicators
    d. Providing a concise presentation of facts and clinical indicators

64. A patient was admitted with heart failure within one week of a heart transplant. Due to the timing, the coder thought the heart failure may indicate a transplant rejection. What action(s) should the coding staff take?

    a. Query the physician.
    b. Assign the codes for the transplant rejection and the heart failure.
    c. Assign only the code for the transplant rejection.
    d. Assign only the code for heart failure.

65. A patient had a normal pregnancy and delivery with loose nuchal cord around neck. Delivery was accompanied by an episiotomy with repair with birth of liveborn male infant. Delivery room record states "no evidence of fetal problem." What is the query opportunity for this record?

    a. Age of the patient
    b. Weeks of gestation/trimester
    c. If there was adequate prenatal care
    d. If the pregnancy was high-risk

Practice Questions

66. A toddler comes into the hospital admitted from the ER with the following: shortness of breath, wheezing, runny nose, and positive RSV test. The final diagnosis was viral infection upon discharge three days later. What condition should the coder query for in this scenario?

    a. Acute bronchiolitis
    b. Acute bronchitis
    c. Croup
    d. Laryngitis

67. While admitted for an exacerbation of COPD, a patient developed swelling in the lower legs and had increasing shortness of breath despite the COPD treatment. An echocardiogram was performed that showed an ejection fraction of 33 percent. A urinalysis showed albuminuria. Breathing treatments continued with the addition of Lasix to the medication regime. In the final diagnostic statement, the physician mentions only the COPD exacerbation. What is the query opportunity for this record?

    a. Coronary artery disease
    b. Acute congestive heart failure
    c. Pleural effusion
    d. Atrial fibrillation

68. Which of the following condition combinations would benefit from a query?

    a. Hypertension and ESRD
    b. Diabetes and polyneuropathy
    c. CHF and hypertension
    d. ESRD and diabetes

69. A patient was admitted with chest pain and shortness of breath. Preliminary lab work indicated nonelevated troponin with LBBB noted on EKG. Patient developed a fever and chills. X-ray finding demonstrated an infiltrate in the left lung. Sputum culture identified *Klebsiella*. The patient slowly improved after antibiotics were administered. Final discharge diagnosis listed as chest pain and patient was sent home on Piperacillin/tazobactam. For which diagnosis does a query opportunity exist for the principal diagnosis?

    a. Gram-negative pneumonia
    b. Aspiration pneumonia
    c. Myocardial infarction
    d. Non-cardiac chest pain

Domain 4 *Regulatory Compliance*

70. Authentication of health record entries means to:

    a. Create facsimiles of documents
    b. Prove authorship of documents
    c. Develop documents
    d. Use a rubber stamp on documents

71. The requirements for documentation and record completion (documents such as history and physicals, discharge summaries, and consultations) as well as penalties for nonadherence must be specified in:

    a. Hospital rules and regulations
    b. Payer guidelines
    c. Medical staff bylaws
    d. Nursing staff policies

72. Generally, data quality is defined as:

    a. Ensuring the greatest amount of data possible is obtained from the medical record
    b. Ensuring the accuracy and completeness of an organization's data
    c. Ensuring accuracy of the data collected for the case-mix index
    d. Ensuring the data for external reporting is optimized

73. The Joint Commission considers management that supports decision making to be important for safety and quality. What kind of management supports decision making?

    a. Resource management
    b. Risk management
    c. Information management
    d. Case management

74. According to Medicare requirements, a history and physical must:

    a. Be coded based on the uniform hospital discharge proposal
    b. Include the patient's weight, height, body mass index, and year of birth
    c. Be completed for each patient no more than 30 days before or 24 hours after admission or registration, but prior to surgery
    d. Discuss the educational plans for the patient including diet, exercise, and plans for smoking cessation

75. Medicare reimbursement depends on all of the following, *except*:

    a. The correct designation of the principal diagnosis
    b. The number of codes that are assigned
    c. The presence or absence of additional codes that represent complications, comorbidities, or major complications/comorbidities
    d. Procedures performed

76. A coder reviews a medical record and determines that a code Medicare has designated as "unacceptable principal diagnosis" is the correct code to assign. What should the coder do?

    a. Assign another code from the history and physical as the principal diagnosis
    b. Assign the code even though the insurer may not pay the claim
    c. Use a comorbidity as the principal diagnosis
    d. Assign a code from the outpatient visit prior to admission

Practice Questions

77. A payer's policy does not cover tetanus injections when provided as a preventive service but will cover them when provided as a postinjury service. If the injection is provided in the emergency department, what part of the claim will need to be modified to indicate the injection was a postinjury service rather than a preventive service?

    a. Diagnosis code
    b. Procedure code
    c. Revenue code
    d. Disposition code

78. Which of the following represents a potential hospital-acquired condition?

    a. Stage 4 pressure ulcer of the coccyx
    b. Foreign body of the skin
    c. Urinary tract infection
    d. Diabetes

79. A 75-year-old patient is admitted for a complex, ventral hernia repair. While in the hospital, the patient slips and falls, suffering a left hip fracture. Will the hip fracture be identified as part of the facility's patient safety indicators (PSI)? Why or why not?

    a. No, the hip fracture is the principal diagnosis and will not be part of the PSI
    b. Yes, the hip fracture is the principal diagnosis and would still be part of the PSI
    c. No, the hip fracture is a secondary diagnosis and therefore, will not be part of the PSI
    d. Yes, the hip fracture is a secondary diagnosis and will be part of the PSI

80. A patient is admitted for treatment of hemophilia with a blood transfusion. The patient had an ABO incompatibility reaction to the transfusion and was taken to the ICU for monitoring and IV saline. The admission is complicated by the development of a pneumonia and the patient's ongoing medical conditions of hypothyroidism and hyperlipidemia, both of which required medication during hospitalization. Breathing treatments continued for the pneumonia and no further transfusions were given. Which condition in the above scenario reflects a hospital-acquired condition?

    a. Hemophilia
    b. Pneumonia
    c. ABO incompatibility
    d. Hypothyroidism

81. An urgent care facility located near a national park treats a significant number of patients with snake bites. Patients receive treatment with antivenom. On occasion, a patient must later be admitted to the hospital. Can the urgent care facility provide the hospital with a list of names of patients treated with snake antivenom?

    a. Only the names of patients who are admitted to the hospital for continuation of care could be provided.
    b. A full list of names could be provided.
    c. No information can be obtained under any circumstances.
    d. A list of patients may be available after consultation with the medical director.

82. The patient was admitted for breast carcinoma in the right breast at two o'clock. This was removed via lumpectomy. An axillary lymph node dissection, performed along with the lumpectomy, identified 1 of 7 lymph nodes positive for carcinoma. One of the patient's neighbors, who works at the hospital, called the coding department to get the patient's diagnosis because she is a cancer survivor herself. The coder should:

    a. Discuss the case with the coworker

    b. Report the incident to hospital security

    c. Give the caller false information

    d. Explain that discussing the case would violate the patient's right to privacy

83. The billing department has requested that copies of patients' final coding summaries with associated code meanings for Medicare be printed remotely in the admission department. Currently, they only request the summaries when there is an unspecified procedure. On previous visits to the admission department, the coding supervisor has found the coding summaries were left on a table near the patient entrance. Of the actions presented here, what would be the best action for the coding supervisor to take?

    a. Comply with the request.

    b. Refuse to undertake this without further explanation.

    c. Ignore the request.

    d. Explain to the billing department supervisor that leaving the coding summary in public view violates the patient's right to privacy.

84. Code sets that are mandated under HIPAA include all of the following *except*:

    a. National Drug Codes

    b. ICD-10-CM and ICD-10-PCS

    c. CPT

    d. Hierarchical Condition Category

85. The electronic transactions and code sets standards are found under which part of HIPAA?

    a. Administrative Simplification

    b. Privacy Rule

    c. Security Rule

    d. Health Information Technology for Economic and Clinical Health Act

86. Determining employee access to patient information should be based on what HIPAA principle?

    a. Medically necessary

    b. Minimum necessary

    c. Nondisclosure

    d. Workforce

Practice Questions

87. A facility's coding policy states that inpatients who undergo open reduction and internal fixation of a fractured femur should be routinely coded with blood loss anemia when there is intraoperative blood loss of 500 cc or more documented in the operative report and the patient has low hemoglobin. Is this correct or incorrect and why?

    a. It is correct to code blood loss anemia because the policy requires it.

    b. It is correct because the clinical signs are documented in the record.

    c. It is incorrect because the patient must also have a blood transfusion in order for blood loss anemia to be coded.

    d. It is incorrect because the physician did not document the blood loss anemia in the progress notes.

88. AHIMA's Standards of Ethical Coding apply to which groups below?

    a. Certified coders

    b. Coding managers

    c. HIM/coding students

    d. Coding auditors

    e. All of the above

    f. A and D only

    g. A and B only

89. At work one day, Mary, who is an outpatient coding professional, overheard another outpatient coder mention that whenever she has a chart to code with a procedure that she is unfamiliar with, she assigns an unlisted CPT code. This allows her to keep up her productivity numbers rather than taking time to research the procedure. What is Mary's ethical responsibility upon learning this information?

    a. None, as she is an outpatient coder and the Code of Ethics applies only to inpatient coders

    b. None, because it is within coding guidelines to assign an unlisted CPT procedure code

    c. Report this to her coding manager as the Code of Ethics requires coders to take steps to correct unethical behavior of colleagues

    d. Report this to the facility's risk manager in order to prevent claim denials

90. A facility recently implemented a computer-assisted coding (CAC) program to assist their coding staff. Since that time, the coding manager has found that one coder, who previously struggled to meet productivity, is now leading the coding staff in productivity. A review shows that he is accepting all CAC suggested codes without validation. Is there an ethical issue here?

    a. Yes, the coding professional is required to utilize CAC as a tool, but not without validating the code choices.

    b. Yes, CAC codes can be assigned only after a coder has independently arrived at the same codes by using a code book.

    c. No, CAC codes are populated based on provider documentation and do not require validation.

    d. No, CAC programs are built by coding professionals, so the auto-suggested codes can automatically be assigned.

91. A retired coding professional has let her CCS credential lapse. However, she is interested in doing some part-time work for a local hospital that only hires credentialed coders. When interviewed, she is asked about her credential and answers that "I have been credentialed as a CCS." Is there an ethical issue with this statement?

    a. No, because it is truthful.

    b. Yes, because the statement does not clearly express that the credential is no longer in effect.

    c. No, because the responsibility for additional information is on the interviewer.

    d. Yes, because the statement is untruthful.

92. Coders at a physician group practice often collaborate on finding the appropriate diagnosis and procedure codes. They do not have access to an encoder, and the books they use are four years old. When they are uncertain about the code selection, they query the physicians. Based on this information, is there anything unethical going on?

    a. Yes; coders should not be collaborating to arrive at diagnosis and procedure codes.

    b. Yes; it is necessary for coders to have access to an encoder to assign codes.

    c. Yes; coders should have current books in order to assign appropriate codes.

    d. Yes; coders should not be querying in a physician office to assign codes.

93. A patient has a principal diagnosis of pneumonia (J18.9) (MS-DRG 195). Which of the following may legitimately change the coding of the pneumonia in accordance with the UHDDS and relevant clinical documentation?

    a. Sputum culture reflects growth of normal flora

    b. Patient has a high fever

    c. Patient is found to have dysphagia with aspiration

    d. Patient has nonproductive cough

94. A patient was admitted to an acute-care facility with a temperature of 102 and atrial fibrillation. The chest x-ray reveals pneumonia with subsequent documentation by the physician of pneumonia in the progress notes and discharge summary. The patient was treated with oral antiarrhythmic medications and IV antibiotics. What is the correct code sequence?

    a. J18.9, I48.91

    b. I48.91, J18.9

    c. It does not matter which is used as the principal diagnosis.

    d. Not enough information is present. Query the physician.

95. The UHDDS definition of principal diagnosis does not apply to the coding of outpatient encounters because:

    a. Assigning codes for signs and symptoms is more relevant for outpatient encounters

    b. Usually there are multiple reasons for the encounter

    c. Short duration of the evaluation does not allow enough time to make an "after study" determination

    d. A preadmission work-up is not available

Practice Questions

96. A patient is admitted for pneumonia. Additionally, the physician has documented the patient has a history of hypertension and diabetes, which require medication (Lisinopril and insulin) while in the hospital, along with a history of migraines and repeated, recent falls. Which of the following diagnoses does not meet the UHDDS definition of additional diagnoses?

    a. I10
    b. Z79.4
    c. R29.6
    d. G43.909

97. In what setting does the UHDDS definition of principal diagnosis not apply?

    a. Hospice
    b. Provider office
    c. Psychiatric hospital
    d. Home health

Multiple Choice Practice Answers

1.	26.	51.	76.
2.	27.	52.	77.
3.	28.	53.	78.
4.	29.	54.	79.
5.	30.	55.	80.
6.	31.	56.	81.
7.	32.	57.	82.
8.	33.	58.	83.
9.	34.	59.	84.
10.	35.	60.	85.
11.	36.	61.	86.
12.	37.	62.	87.
13.	38.	63.	88.
14.	39.	64.	89.
15.	40.	65.	90.
16.	41.	66.	91.
17.	42.	67.	92.
18.	43.	68.	93.
19.	44.	69.	94.
20.	45.	70.	95.
21.	46.	71.	96.
22.	47.	72.	97.
23.	48.	73.	
24.	49.	74.	
25.	50.	75.	

CCS

PRACTICE CASE STUDIES

Practice Case Studies

Note: Review the Guidelines for Coding the CCS Exam Preparation Case Studies in the Introduction of this book.

AMBULATORY CASE—PATIENT 1

FACE SHEET

DATE OF ADMISSION: 4/5   **DATE OF DISCHARGE:** 4/5

SEX: Male   **AGE:** 37   **DISCHARGE DISPOSITION:** Home

ADMISSION DIAGNOSIS: Left inguinal hernia

DISCHARGE DIAGNOSIS: Same

PROCEDURES: Left inguinal herniorrhaphy with excision of lipoma of spermatic cord

HISTORY AND PHYSICAL EXAMINATION—PATIENT 1

ADMITTED: 4/5

HISTORY OF PRESENT ILLNESS: The patient has been well until several months ago when he began to have pain when lifting.

PAST MEDICAL HISTORY: The patient has no other significant medical or surgical history.

SOCIAL HISTORY: Does not use alcohol or tobacco

ALLERGIES: No known allergies

MEDICATIONS: None

REVIEW OF SYSTEMS:

    SKIN: Warm and dry, mucous membranes moist

    HEENT: Essentially normal

    LUNGS: Clear to percussion and auscultation

    HEART: Normal, regular rhythm

    ABDOMEN: Normal

    GENITALIA: Palpable mass in inguinal canal

    RECTAL: Normal

    EXTREMITIES: No edema

    NEUROLOGIC: Deep tendon reflexes normal

IMPRESSION: Left inguinal hernia

PLAN: Surgical repair of inguinal hernia

PROGRESS NOTES—PATIENT 1

DATE	NOTE
4/5	Nursing: Betadine scrub performed, patient anxious to get surgery over; preoperative medications given as ordered.
4/5	Attending MD: Brief op note Dx: Left inguinal hernia Px: Left inguinal herniorrhaphy Anes: Local plus sedation Complications: None
4/5	Attending MD: No bleeding; patient okay for discharge.

OPERATIVE REPORT—PATIENT 1

DATE: 4/5

PREOPERATIVE DIAGNOSIS: Left direct inguinal hernia

POSTOPERATIVE DIAGNOSIS: Left direct inguinal hernia

OPERATION: Left inguinal herniorrhaphy

ANESTHESIA: Local plus sedation

OPERATIVE INDICATIONS: A wide mouth direct sac was present in the lower inguinal canal. A lipoma of the cord was present, but no indirect sac.

OPERATIVE PROCEDURE: Under local anesthesia consisting of the equivalent of 19 cc of 1% Xylocaine and 8 cc of 0.5% Marcaine, the abdomen was prepared with Betadine and sterilely draped. A left inguinal incision was made and carried down through subcutaneous tissues to the aponeurosis of the external oblique, which was opened from the external ring to a point over the internal ring. Flaps were cleaned in both directions. The nerve was retracted inferiorly. The cord structures were separated from the surrounding at the level of the pubic tubercle and retracted with a Penrose drain. Cremaster over the cord was opened and a search made for an indirect sac. None was found. Lipoma of the cord was dissected free and clamped at its base and excised. The base was ligated with 00 chromic catgut. Additional cremasteric muscles were divided and ligated with 00 chromic catgut. The direct sac was further dissected down to its base and inverted as the defect was closed by approximating transversus to transversus with a running suture of 00 Vicryl. The floor of the canal was then closed by approximating the internal oblique to the shelving portion of the inguinal ligament with multiple sutures of 0 Ethibond. The external oblique aponeurosis was then reclosed with 0 Ethibond, leaving the cord and nerve in the subcutaneous position. Several sutures of 0 Ethibond were also placed above the emergence of the cord at the internal ring. Subcutaneous tissues were then approximated with 3-0 Vicryl and after irrigation skin was closed with skin clips. The patient tolerated the procedure well and was sent to the recovery room in good condition.

PATHOLOGY REPORT—PATIENT 1

DATE SPECIMEN SUBMITTED: 4/5

SPECIMEN: Lipoma of cord

CLINICAL DATA:

GROSS DESCRIPTION: The specimen is submitted as lipoma of cord. It consists of a single irregularly shaped fragment of fatty tissue that is 8.0 × 4.0 × 1.5 cm. It is covered with a thin membrane.

MICROSCOPIC DESCRIPTION:

DIAGNOSIS: Lipomatous tissue of left spermatic cord

PHYSICIAN'S ORDERS—PATIENT 1

DATE	ORDER
4/5	Attending MD: Admit to same-day surgery Betadine scrub ×3 Preop May take own meds
4/5	Anesthesia note: Continue NPO Demerol 50 mg IM 1½ hr Preop Vistaril 50 mg IM 1½ hr Preop Atropine 0.4 mg IM 1½ hr Preop
4/5	Attending MD: VITAL SIGNS Q. 15 MIN UNTIL STABLE Regular diet Darvocet-N-100 q. 4 hrs p.r.n. pain Discharge to home when stable

LABORATORY REPORTS—PATIENT 1

HEMATOLOGY

DATE: 4/5

Specimen	Results	Normal
WBC	6.83	4.3–11.0
RBC	4.57	4.5–5.9
HGB	13.7	13.5–17.5
HCT	43	41–52
MCV	87.0	80–100
MCHC	35	31–57
PLT	300	150–400

AUTO DIFFERENTIAL—PATIENT 1

DATE: 4/5

Specimen	Results	Normal Values
NEUT	68.3	40.0–74.0
LYMPH	20	19.0–48.0
MONO	5.6	3.4–9.0
EOS	5.6	0.0–7.0
BASO	0.6	0.0–1.5
LUC	3.8	0.0–4.0

URINALYSIS—PATIENT 1

DATE: 4/5

Test	Result	Ref Range
SP GRAVITY	1.017	1.005–1.035
PH	6	5–7
PROT	TRACE	NEG
GLUC	NONE	NEG
KETONES	NONE	NEG
BILI	NONE	NEG
BLOOD	TRACE	NEG
NITRATES	NONE	NEG
RBCS	NONE	NEG
WBCS	NONE	NEG

Practice Case Studies

RADIOLOGY REPORT—PATIENT 1

DATE: 4/5

DIAGNOSIS: Inguinal hernia

EXAMINATION: Chest x-ray

Heart size and shape are acceptable. The lung fields are clear and the pulmonary vascular pattern is unremarkable. There is no free fluid and the trachea remains midline.

Choose the correct principal diagnosis code.

- a. K40.10
- b. K40.21
- c. K40.30
- d. K40.41
- e. K40.90

Choose the correct secondary diagnosis code(s).

- a. D17.30
- b. D17.39
- c. D17.4
- d. D17.5
- e. D17.6
- f. D17.9
- g. D29.31
- h. D29.32
- i. D29.4
- j. None apply

Choose the correct procedure code(s).

- a. 49491-50
- b. 49495-LT
- c. 49500-RT
- d. 49505-LT
- e. 49525
- f. 49650
- g. 49651
- h. 55500-25
- i. 55520-59
- j. 55540-27

AMBULATORY CASE—PATIENT 2

DIAGNOSIS: Low back pain, lumbar radiculopathy with chronic pain syndrome

HISTORY: This is an 18-year-old white female with low back pain and lumbar radicular pain for epidural steroid injection. The patient had an epidural approximately three weeks ago with approximately 30% improvement. The patient is agreeable for an additional epidural steroid injection for pain management.

PROCEDURE: Epidural steroid injection under C-arm guidance via caudal approach and epidurogram. The patient was transferred to the operating room and placed in the prone position. Under MAC anesthesia her low back and sacral areas were sterilely prepped and draped. Local 1% lidocaine was applied with a #23-gauge needle through the skin and surrounding tissues of the sacral hiatus. Then a #17-gauge Epimed needle was inserted percutaneously through the sacral hiatus into the epidural space. This was confirmed via lateral view of the C-arm. Then under AP fluoroscopy, a #18-gauge Epimed catheter was guided to the mid L3-L4 area of the nerve root in the midline. Next, 2 cc of Isovue dye were injected, which showed good bilateral spread in the epidural space. A solution of 6 cc of normal saline, 80 mg of Depo-Medrol and 2 cc of 1% lidocaine was partially deposited at the L3-L4 nerve root. The catheter was then moved down to the L4-L5 nerve root in the midline of the epidural space. An additional 1 cc of Isovue dye was injected, which showed good bilateral spread. An additional one third of local anesthetic Depo-Medrol solution was deposited at the L4-L5 nerve root. The catheter was then moved down to the L5-S1 nerve root and in the midline. Another 1 cc of Isovue dye was injected, which confirmed good bilateral spread and highlighting of the L5-S1 nerve roots bilateral. The remaining local anesthetic Depo-Medrol solution was deposited at the L5-S1 nerve root. The catheter and needle were then pulled intact and the patient was transferred to the recovery room in satisfactory condition.

IMPRESSION: Low back pain, lumbar radiculopathy. This is the patient's second epidural steroid injection.

FOLLOW-UP: After seeing improvement in the next 24 to 48 hours and repeat injection if necessary.

Choose the correct principal diagnosis code.

a. G89.0
b. G89.18
c. G89.4
d. G90.521
e. R52

Choose the correct secondary diagnosis code(s).

a. M54.16
b. M54.17
c. M54.30
d. M54.31
e. M54.32
f. M54.40
g. M54.41
h. M54.42
i. M54.5
j. None apply

Practice Case Studies

Choose the correct procedure code(s).

   a. 62270-RT
   b. 62272
   c. 62322
   d. 62323
   e. 62324
   f. 62325-50
   g. 62326
   h. 62327
   i. 62328-RT, LT
   j. 62329

AMBULATORY RECORD—PATIENT 3

DATE: 8/12/20XX

SURGERY RECORD:

PATIENT HISTORY: This patient is seen today to insert an intrathecal pump for pain management due to ductal carcinoma of the upper and lower quadrants of left breast metastatic to the vertebrae of the spine. She previously underwent modified radical mastectomy within the last month and a half with general anesthesia and had no adverse effects. No other surgical history is given. No known allergies, no current medications. Review of systems is normal.

Following preoperative evaluation and discussion with the patient, local anesthesia was used to implant an intrathecal programmable pump surgically placed and attached to a previously placed catheter. The patient tolerated the procedure well. There were no adverse effects of anesthesia.

Choose the correct principal diagnosis code.

a. G89.18
b. G89.3
c. G89.4
d. G90.521
e. R52

Choose the correct secondary diagnosis code(s).

a. C50.212
b. C50.312
c. C50.412
d. C50.512
e. C50.612
f. C50.812
g. C77.3
h. C79.51
i. C79.9
j. None apply

Practice Case Studies

Choose the correct procedure code(s).

a. 62324
b. 62325
c. 62326
d. 62327
e. 62350
f. 62351
g. 62355
h. 62360
i. 62361
j. 62362

Practice Case Studies

AMBULATORY RECORD—PATIENT 4

PREOPERATIVE DIAGNOSIS: Reflex sympathetic dystrophy, left knee

POSTOPERATIVE DIAGNOSIS: Reflex sympathetic dystrophy, left knee

OPERATION: Left lumbar sympathetic block with C-arm

ANESTHESIA: Local

INDICATIONS:

This 43-year-old female has a 7-month history of left knee pain. She says that even a light touch appears to be exquisitely painful. She has had surgery to clear scar tissue.

PROCEDURE DESCRIPTION:

The patient was placed on the x-ray lucent gurney in the right lateral decubitus position. The back was prepped with Betadine, and the midline spinous processes were marked. A line was drawn 6 to 7 cm lateral to that midline on the left. L2 was identified using the C-arm and lateral projections, and lidocaine was infiltrated at the skin. The 22-gauge, 6-inch Chiba needle was advanced down to and off the body of L2, and loss of resistance was obtained with a glass syringe. Renografin-60 was injected and showed a good distribution. So 15 cc of bupivacaine 0.5% without epinephrine was injected, plus Depo-Medrol 40 mg. The needle was withdrawn.

Then lidocaine was infiltrated on the 6- to 7-cm line at L4. I advanced the 22-gauge, 6-inch needle off the body of L4, but the Renografin-60 distribution appeared not to be adequate. Another wheal was raised at the L3 level, and the needle was advanced down to and off the body of L3. A loss of resistance was obtained with a glass syringe, followed by Renografin-60. This time, the distribution was excellent, and bupivacaine 0.5% without epinephrine = 15 cc was injected. She was left on her side for 25 minutes. After 10 minutes, she had a noticeably warmer left foot and ankle. The skin coloration of the left leg was normal.

Choose the correct principal diagnosis code.

   a. G89.0
   b. G89.28
   c. G89.51
   d. G90.522
   e. R52

Practice Case Studies

Choose the correct secondary diagnosis code(s).

a. G89.0
b. G89.11
c. G89.21
d. M25.561
e. M25.562
f. M25.569
g. M79.661
h. M79.662
i. M79.669
j. None apply

Choose the correct procedure code(s).

a. 62324-LT
b. 62326
c. 64435-50
d. 64490
e. 64491
f. 64493-LT
g. 64494-59
h. 64520-LT
i. 64520-59-LT
j. 77003

Practice Case Studies

EMERGENCY DEPARTMENT RECORD—PATIENT 5

DATE OF ADMISSION: 4/1   **DATE OF DISCHARGE:** 4/1

HISTORY (PROBLEM FOCUSED):

HISTORY OF PRESENT ILLNESS: This is a 16-year-old African American female with pierced ears who, while removing her sweater, got it caught on her earring, accidentally pulling the earring out and lacerating her left ear lobe.

PAST MEDICAL HISTORY: The patient has a history of childhood asthma that has not occurred for several years.

ALLERGIES: Penicillin

CHRONIC MEDICATIONS: None

REVIEW OF SYSTEMS: The patient has been well.

PHYSICAL EXAMINATION (PROBLEM FOCUSED):

GENERAL APPEARANCE: This is a well-nourished 16-year-old black female in no apparent distress. HEENT normal except for 2 cm laceration of left earlobe. Neck veins flat at 40-degree angle. No nodes felt in the neck, carotids, or groin. Carotid pulsations are normal. No bruits heard in the neck. Chest clear on percussion and auscultation. Heart is not enlarged. No thrills or murmurs. Rhythm is regular. BP 130/80. Liver and spleen not palpable. No masses felt in the abdomen. No ascites noted. No edema of the extremities. Pulses in the feet are good.

IMPRESSION: Laceration of left ear lobe

PLAN: Suture laceration of left ear lobe

TREATMENT: Following infiltration of the areas with Xylocaine, the laceration was closed with 2-0 Vicryl. Two suture kits were used.

DISCHARGE DIAGNOSIS: Ear lobe laceration of left ear

INSTRUCTIONS ON DISCHARGE: Demerol by mouth 50 mg every 6 hours as needed for pain. Biaxin 500 mg PO b.i.d. for 10 days. Follow up with surgical clinic in 7 days.

Emergency Department Evaluation and Management Mapping

The following are the number of acuity points needed to assign a particular level of CPT code:

Level 1 = 1–20

Level 2 = 21–35

Level 3 = 36–47

Level 4 = 48–60

Level 5 = > 61

Critical Care > 61 with constant physician attendance

CPT Codes

Level 1 = 99281   99281–25 with procedure/laboratory/radiology

Level 2 = 99282   99282–25 with procedure/laboratory/radiology

Level 3 = 99283   99283–25 with procedure/laboratory/radiology

Level 4 = 99284   99284–25 with procedure/laboratory/radiology

Level 5 = 99285   99285–25 with procedure/laboratory/radiology

Practice Case Studies

Emergency Department Acuity Points					
	5	10	15	20	25
Number of Meds Given	0–2	3–5	6–7	8–9	>10
Extent of Hx	Brief	PF	EPF	Detail	Comprehensive
Extent of Exam	Brief	PF	EPF	Detail	Comprehensive
Number of Tests Ordered	0–1	2–3	4–5	6–7	>8
Number of Supplies Used	1	2–3	4–5	6–7	>8

Choose the correct principal diagnosis code.

a. S01.312A
b. S01.321A
c. S01.331A
d. S01.342A
e. S01.352A

Choose the correct secondary diagnosis code(s).

a. H92.01
b. H92.02
c. H92.09
d. H92.12
e. J45.20
f. J45.41
g. J45.909
h. R01.1
i. R19.15
j. None apply

Choose the correct procedure code(s).

a. 12001
b. 12002
c. 12011
d. 12013
e. 12031
f. 12041
g. 12042
h. 99282-27
i. 99283-25
j. 99284

INPATIENT RECORD—PATIENT 6

DISCHARGE SUMMARY

DATE OF ADMISSION: 11/30   **DATE OF DISCHARGE:** 12/4

DISCHARGE DIAGNOSIS: Fracture of neck of right femur

ADMISSION HISTORY: The patient is a 78-year-old male who fell on the day of admission and sustained a fracture of the neck of his right femur. The patient was admitted for a medical evaluation prior to surgical intervention.

COURSE IN HOSPITAL: Medical evaluation was obtained on admission. Patient was taken to the operating room, where an open reduction and internal fixation of the fracture of the right femur was performed. Postoperative course was complicated by urinary retention, which necessitated the placement of an indwelling Foley catheter. He was discharged with the catheter in place. The patient was ambulatory, nonweight bearing with a walker at the time of discharge.

INSTRUCTIONS ON DISCHARGE: The patient is instructed to follow up with my office in 3 days to remove staples and to begin outpatient physical therapy tomorrow. Home health services will follow this patient. Pain medications: Darvocet N 100, one tablet every 4 hours as needed for pain.

Practice Case Studies

HISTORY AND PHYSICAL EXAMINATION—PATIENT 6

ADMITTED: 11/30

REASON FOR ADMISSION: Right hip pain following a fall

HISTORY OF PRESENT ILLNESS: The patient is a 78-year-old male who fell on the day of admission and sustained a fracture of the neck of his right femur. The patient was admitted for a medical evaluation prior to surgical intervention.

PAST MEDICAL HISTORY: The patient has had multiple medical problems including gastric ulcer, congestive heart failure, diverticulosis, degenerative joint disease, arteriosclerotic coronary artery disease, and mitral regurgitation.

ALLERGIES: None

CHRONIC MEDICATIONS: Lanoxin 0.125 mg, Mon. Wed., and Fri., Lasix 40 mg q. a.m., Lasix 40 mg q. p.m., Colace 200 mg q. a.m., Metamucil one teaspoon b.i.d., Zestril 10 mg every day, Zantac 150 mg PO b.i.d., nitroglycerin 0.4 mg. PRN for chest pain, Celebrex 100 mg PO b.i.d. for degenerative joint disease, Razadyne for dementia.

SOCIAL HISTORY: The patient is widowed with 3 children and 7 grandchildren. The patient is a nondrinker and nonsmoker.

REVIEW OF SYSTEMS: The patient has been in usual health until the day prior to admission when he fell. There has been no change in bladder and bowel functioning. Cognitively, he has dementia.

PHYSICAL EXAMINATION: BP is 170/90, pulse 80 and regular. The patient is an elderly, thin, somewhat deaf male. His pupils are small and reactive to light. The pharynx is benign. The jugular pulse is distended but filled from above. He has no supraclavicular adenopathy. His chest is clear. On palpation the pericardium was located in his anterior axillary line with a palpable thrill. On auscultation he had a harsh grade III/VI apical systolic murmur that radiated to the apex and faintly to the lower left sternal edge. He had a soft diastolic flow murmur. His abdomen was somewhat tense without organomegaly. He had minimal peripheral edema.

CONSULTATION—PATIENT 6

DATE: 11/30

CHIEF COMPLAINT: Pain in hip

REVIEW OF SYSTEMS: The patient has been in usual health until the day prior to admission when he fell. The patient is experiencing a little more shortness of breath than usual. The patient is unsure if he felt dizzy before falling.

PHYSICAL EXAMINATION: This is an elderly, moderately nourished white male. HEENT reveals nothing abnormal. There is no adenopathy. His chest is clear with loud grade III/VI pansystolic murmur. Examination of the abdomen reveals no masses or tenderness. He had minimal peripheral edema with one leg appearing shorter than the other. Distal circulation and sensation are normal.

IMPRESSION:

History of gastric ulcer

Congestive heart failure

Diverticulosis

Degenerative joint disease

Arteriosclerotic coronary artery disease

Mitral regurgitation

PLAN: D/C NSAIDs for now in light of GI history. Maintain low residue diet in light of diverticulosis. The patient is cleared for surgery.

Practice Case Studies

PROGRESS NOTES—PATIENT 6

DATE	NOTE
11/30	Patient admitted for medical evaluation prior to ORIF. The patient is somewhat confused about the events surrounding the fall. At present he offers no other complaint. The patient currently has Bucks traction in place. If cleared for surgery, patient is scheduled for tomorrow at 1:00 p.m.
12/1	The patient is resting quietly. Medication adequate to alleviate pain in extremity.
6:30 a.m.	Operative consent signed following obtaining informed consent for surgery. All questions from patient and family answered. **PREOP DX:** Fracture of right femur
6:30 p.m.	**POSTOP DX:** Same **OPERATION:** Open reduction, internal fixation, femoral neck fracture, right hip **ANESTHESIA:** Spinal and general **COMPLICATIONS:** None Patient sleeping. Dressings intact, hemovac in place.
8:00 p.m.	House Physician called to see patient due to inability to void. The patient appears to have a postop complication of urinary retention. Will place Foley catheter.
12/2	Events of last night noted. Will request that patient get OOB and begin physical therapy. Hemovac in place draining small amount. Patient not complaining of pain. H&H looks good. Lytes fine.
12/3	Patient has been ambulating well. Patient minimally confused due to senile dementia. Neurovascular status good. Appetite good. Dressing intact, incision healing well, no redness or inflammation.
12/4	Patient up with assistance and ambulating using walker. Incision healing well. Discharge with indwelling Foley. Home health services to assist patient following discharge. Ready for discharge today.

PHYSICIAN'S ORDERS—PATIENT 6

DATE	ORDER
11/30	Admit to floor
	NPO after midnight
	Continue present meds:
	Lanoxin 0.125 mg, q.d.
	Lasix 40 mg q. a.m. and p.m.
	Colace 200 mg q. a.m.
	Metamucil one teaspoon b.i.d.
	Zantac 150 mg po b.i.d.
	Celebrex 100 mg po b.i.d. for DJD
	Prep for hip surgery
	Medical Consult for surgical clearance
	4 lb Bucks traction to continue
	Demerol 50 mg q. 3 to 4 hours
	Darvocet N 100 q. 3 to 4 hours
	Cross match 3 units of blood
	Low sodium, low-fat diet
	Dig level in a.m.
	H&H and electrolytes
12/1	Preop Meds
	Hold Dig this a.m.
	Ancef 1 g on call to OR
	Postop Meds
	Run D5W 1,000 cc q. 12 hrs
	Demerol 500 mg q. 3 to 4 hrs p.r.n. pain
	Darvocet N 100 q. 3 to 4 hours
	Hct and Hgb at 9:00 p.m. and in a.m.
	Electrolytes in a.m.
	Ancef 500 mg IV q. 6 hrs × 4 doses
	X-ray hip in a.m.
	Ice on hip
	Up in chair following x-ray
	Begin physical therapy tomorrow
	Insert Foley catheter
12/2	Consult home health services for discharge needs. Continue pain meds. Get patient OOB for ambulation with walker.
12/3	D/C IV
12/4	D/C patient. Home health services to follow.

Practice Case Studies

OPERATIVE REPORT—PATIENT 6

DATE: 12/1

PREOPERATIVE DIAGNOSIS: Fracture of right femoral neck

POSTOPERATIVE DIAGNOSIS: Same

OPERATION: Open reduction and internal fixation of fracture right femoral neck

ANESTHESIA: Spinal and general

OPERATIVE INDICATIONS:

OPERATIVE PROCEDURE: The patient was given Ancef 1 g IV 30 minutes prior to the procedure for endocarditis/surgical prophylaxis. The patient was administered a spinal anesthesia and then placed on the fracture table in traction. X-rays revealed satisfactory position and alignment of the fracture site. The right hip was prepped with Betadine scrub and Betadine solution and draped in a sterile fashion. A straight incision was made over the lateral aspect of the right hip and carried through the subcutaneous tissue, then tensor fascia lata and vastus lateralis muscles so that the fracture could be reduced and fixation devices utilized. The lateral shaft of the femur was exposed subperiosteally. A guide wire was then placed into the neck and head of the femur and x-rays revealed a slightly inferior position. The new guide wire was obtained in satisfactory position. The lateral shaft, neck, and head of the femur were then drilled to a depth of 85 mm with the drill. An 85-mm, 140-degree and 5-degree compression nail were then inserted over which a 140-degree angle 4-hole side plate was then inserted. A compression screw was then applied after the key was inserted. The side plate was then fixed to the shaft of the femur with four screws. X-rays revealed satisfactory position and alignment of the neck fracture fragments and the fixation device. The wound was then well irrigated. A large hemovac drain was inserted and brought out through a separate stab wound incision. The wound was closed with a continuous #000 Vicryl suture in the vastus lateralis and tensor fascia lata layers. The subcutaneous tissue was closed with interrupted #000 Vicryl sutures and the skin was closed with staples. A compression dressing was applied. The patient tolerated the procedure well and there were no operative complications. Patient was returned to the recovery room in satisfactory condition.

LABORATORY REPORTS—PATIENT 6

HEMATOLOGY

DATE: 11/30

Specimen	Results	Normal Values
WBC	9.9	4.3–11.0
RBC	5.0	4.5–5.9
HGB	14.0	13.5–17.5
HCT	45	41–52
MCV	89	80–100
MCHC	33.9	31–57
PLT	Adequate	150–450

HEMATOLOGY— PATIENT 6

DATE: 12/1

Specimen	Results	Normal Values
WBC	7.7	4.3–11.0
RBC	4.4 L	4.5–5.9
HGB	13.2 L	13.5–17.5
HCT	41	41–52
MCV	89	80–100
MCHC	33.9	31–57
PLT	Adequate	150–450

HEMATOLOGY— PATIENT 6

DATE: 12/1

Specimen	Results	Normal Values
WBC	8.0	4.3–11.0
RBC	4.5	4.5–5.9
HGB	13.7	13.5–17.5
HCT	42	41–52
MCV	89	80–100
MCHC	33.9	31–57
PLT	Adequate	150–450

Practice Case Studies

CHEMISTRY— PATIENT 6

DATE: 11/30

Specimen	Results	Normal Values
GLUC	97	70–110
BUN	12	8–25
CREAT	1.0	0.5–1.5
NA	138	136–146
K	4.0	3.5–5.5
CL	109	95–110
CO_2	33 H	24–32
CA	9.1	8.4–10.5
PHOS	3.0	2.5–4.4
MG	2.0	1.6–3.0
T BILI	1.0	0.2–1.2
D BILI	0.4	0.0–0.5
PROTEIN	7.0	6.0–8.0
ALBUMIN	5.4	5.0–5.5
AST	36	0–40
ALT	44	30–65
GCT	70	15–85
LD	110	100–190
ALK PHOS	114	50–136
URIC ACID	6.0	2.2–7.7
CHOL	165	0–200
TRIG	140	10–160

CHEMISTRY— PATIENT 6

DATE: 12/1

Specimen	Results	Normal Values
GLUC	97	70–110
BUN	12	8–25
CREAT	1.0	0.5–1.5
NA	134 L	136–146
K	5.6 H	3.5–5.5
CL	109	95–110
CO_2	33 H	24–32
CA	9.1	8.4–10.5
PHOS	3.0	2.5–4.4
MG	2.0	1.6–3.0
T BILI	1.0	0.2–1.2
D BILI	0.4	0.0–0.5
PROTEIN	7.0	6.0–8.0
ALBUMIN	5.4	5.0–5.5
AST	36	0–40
ALT	44	30–65
GGT	70	15–85
LD	110	100–190
ALK PHOS	114	50–136
URIC ACID	6.0	2.2–7.7
CHOL	165	0–200
TRIG	140	10–160

RADIOLOGY REPORT— PATIENT 6

DATE: 11/30

RIGHT HIP AND FEMUR: A displaced femoral neck fracture is noted with a mild degree of varus angulation. The adjacent skeletal structures are normal. The right femur is intact beyond the neck. There is vascular calcification.

CHEST, SUPINE: There is no gross evidence of acute inflammatory disease or congestive heart failure.

IMPRESSION: Femur and hip; slightly angulated, femoral neck fracture; chest; no acute disease.

Practice Case Studies

RADIOLOGY REPORT—PATIENT 6

DATE: 12/2

DIAGNOSIS: *RIGHT HIP AND FEMUR.* The displaced, femoral neck fracture has been surgically corrected. The adjacent skeletal structures are normal.

IMPRESSION: The fracture is maintained with an orthopedic device.

Choose the correct principal diagnosis code.

- a. S72.001A
- b. S72.009A
- c. S72.031A
- d. S72.043A
- e. S72.099A

Choose the correct secondary diagnosis code(s).

- a. F03.90
- b. I25.10
- c. I34.0
- d. I50.9
- e. K57.90
- f. M19.90
- g. N99.89
- h. R33.8
- i. Z87.11
- j. None apply

Choose the correct procedure code(s).

- a. 0QS204Z
- b. 0QS345Z
- c. 0QS604Z
- d. 0QS73CZ
- e. 0QSB06Z
- f. 0T9030Z
- g. 0T9640Z
- h. 0T9700Z
- i. 0T9840Z
- j. 0T9B70Z

SAME-DAY SURGERY RECORD—PATIENT 7

DATE OF ADMISSION: 1/29　　　**DATE OF DISCHARGE:** 1/29

DISCHARGE DIAGNOSIS: Torn lateral meniscus of the right knee; torn anterior cruciate ligament of the right knee

ADMISSION HISTORY: The patient is a 17-year-old male, who injured his knee in a surfing accident and for this reason was taken for arthroscopic evaluation and treatment.

COURSE IN HOSPITAL: The patient was taken to the OR where a resection of tear of the lateral meniscus posterior horn and reconstruction of the anterior cruciate ligament using patellar tendon graft was performed. The patient was then discharged and asked to return in 1 week.

INSTRUCTIONS ON DISCHARGE:

Levaquin 500 mg by mouth, 1 per day

Tylox 1–2 capsules as needed for pain

Follow-up appointment in 1 week

HISTORY AND PHYSICAL EXAMINATION—PATIENT 7

DATE: 1/29

HISTORY OF PRESENT ILLNESS: This is a 17-year-old male active in several sports. He injured the knee while surfing.

PAST MEDICAL HISTORY: The patient has no other health problems.

ALLERGIES: None known

CHRONIC MEDICATIONS: None

FAMILY HISTORY: Noncontributory

PHYSICAL EXAMINATION: Reveals a well-developed, well-nourished white male in no apparent distress. HEENT reveals nothing abnormal. Chest was clear to auscultation and percussion. Heart sounds were normal with no murmurs. Examination of the abdomen reveals no masses or tenderness. Examination of the genitals was not done. Examination of the extremities reveals a scar on the left knee with swelling of the joint. Distal sensation and circulation were normal.

IMPRESSION: Torn lateral meniscus of the right knee; torn anterior cruciate ligament of the right knee.

PLAN:

1. Resection of tear of the lateral meniscus posterior horn
2. Reconstruction of the anterior cruciate ligament using patellar tendon graft

Practice Case Studies

PROGRESS NOTES—PATIENT 7

DATE	NOTE
1/29	Admit to Same-Day Surgery unit
	Prep for surgery
	Betadine scrub right leg
	Demerol 100 mg IM 1 hr preop
	Versed 5 mg IM 1 hr preop
	Postop Orders:
	Demerol 75 mg. PRN pain 1 dose
	Tylox 1 to 2 PO q. 4 hr
	Levaquin 500 mg PO postop
	D/C when stable as per discharge criteria

PHYSICIAN'S ORDERS—PATIENT 7

DATE	ORDER
1/29	Patient admitted for surgical and diagnostic arthroscopy
	Brief OP Note

PREOP DX: Torn lateral meniscus of the right knee; torn anterior cruciate ligament of the right knee

POSTOP DX: Torn lateral meniscus of the right knee; torn anterior cruciate ligament of the right knee

OPERATION:

1. Resection of tear of the lateral meniscus posterior horn
2. Reconstruction of the anterior cruciate ligament using patellar tendon graft

ANES: General

Good circulation and sensation. Will encourage patient to ambulate with splint and crutches.

Discharge when stable. Follow up in one week with my office.

DISCHARGE MEDICATIONS:

1. Levaquin 500 mg by mouth, one per day
2. Tylox 1–2 capsules as needed for pain

OPERATIVE REPORT—PATIENT 7

PREOPERATIVE DIAGNOSIS: Torn lateral meniscus of the right knee; torn anterior cruciate ligament of the right knee

POSTOPERATIVE DIAGNOSIS: Torn lateral meniscus of the right knee; torn anterior cruciate ligament of the right knee

OPERATION:

1. Resection of tear of the lateral meniscus posterior horn
2. Reconstruction of the anterior cruciate ligament using patellar tendon graft

ANESTHESIA: General

CLINICAL HISTORY: This is a 17-year-old male who sustained an injury to his right knee during a surfing accident. He wished to have the following procedure done.

Tourniquet was used for one hour, 50 minutes

PROCEDURE DESCRIPTION: The patient was placed under general anesthesia. Airway was maintained by Dr. Spears, as the right lower limb was manipulated and found to have a positive Lachman, a positive drawer test, and a trace pivot shift. The left knee was also examined and found to have the same findings.

The knee was prepped with a gel prep, draped with the limb free. Tourniquet was applied to the thigh but not elevated to begin with. The procedure done first was a diagnostic arthroscopy, and, during this, we found that the anterior cruciate ligament was torn away from the wall lateral femoral condyle. It was quite lax as well. Attention was turned to the lateral compartment where the initial look at the lateral cartilage showed that it was fine. But on probing underneath the surface of the posterior horn, there was a partial tear but without any instability. The tear extended through the cartilage 50% to 75%. Because of this, this portion was resected back to normal cartilage, removing the torn segment. This was in an area that was not vascular.

Attention was then turned to the anterior cruciate ligament which was resected. Using a shaver, all the soft tissue was removed from around and up into the notch. A bur was used to enlarge the notch superiorly, into the lateral side and into the depth of the notch to the over-the-top position that was clearly delineated.

The first part of the arthroscopy was terminated. The tourniquet was elevated. Then an incision was made from the mid patella to the tibial tubercle, with dissection carried down to the patellar tendon. The middle third of the patellar tendon was harvested with bone graft from tibia and fibula which was sized to a 10-rom tunnel size. Two threads were placed in the femoral portion and one in the tibial portion, and the femoral portion marked at the interface between the bone and the tendon. The small saw was used to cut the bone graft from both the tibia and the patella. The patellar defect was filled with bone graft and closed. The guide for the tibial tunnel was then put in place, measuring about 55 degrees. This was placed just in front of the posterior tibial tendon and in the mid portion of the slope of the tibial spine. The guide wire was put in place, found to be satisfactory, and a 10-rom channel was reamed. The over-the-top positioning was put into placed with a guidewire. This was in the eleven o'clock for the right knee. The bulldog cannulated reamer was used, and a footprint was established. Probing revealed there to be a millimeter of bone posterior to this. This was reamed up to 30 mm in size for the graft plus 5 rom. The guidewire was removed. The eccentric guide was put into place, and a notch made. Then the two-pin passer was passed through the eccentric guide, and then the guide was removed. The exit of the two-pin passer was in a proper place on the anterolateral thigh. A guidewire was used to put in place in the two-pin passer, and the graft was passed up into the channel and seemed to fit well. A biodegradable screw was used, but the first one did not cut properly and had to be replaced after tapping the spot for the screw.

Practice Case Studies

OPERATIVE REPORT—PATIENT 7

A second biodegradable screw was put up in place. This was approximately 25 mm × 9 mm. The position and tightness were excellent, and drawer test at this point was trace, as was the Lachman. There was no impingement of the graft with extension, and no change in the length. The screw for the tibia was put into place over a guidewire, and this was an 8 × 25 tibial screw. This again was quite tight, and the Lachman test was just a trace positive.

The joint and the wound were irrigated with arthroscopic fluid, and subcutaneous tissues were closed with 2-0 Vicryl. The skin was closed with 4-0 nylon, as was each of the ports. The incision plus the ports were all injected with 0.25% Marcaine with epinephrine. The patient was given 30 mg of Toradol. Dressing was applied of Xeroform gauze, 4 × 4s, Kerlix, Ace wrap, and then the patient's brace which was a Bledsoe brace.

He tolerated the procedure well with a tourniquet time of 1 hour 50 minutes. Blood loss was nil. He will be sent home on Lortab. He will return to the office on Friday for a dressing change. He will be contacted tomorrow.

PHYSICIAN'S ORDERS—PATIENT 7

DATE	ORDER
4/1/20XX	Attending MD: Admit to same-day surgery Betadine scrub ×3 Preop May take own meds Lasix 20 mg now
4/1/20XX	Anesthesia Note: Continue NPO Demerol 50 mg IM 1½ hr Preop Vistaril 50 mg IM 1½ hr Preop Atropine 0.4 mg IM 1½ hr Preop
4/1/20XX	Attending MD: Vital signs q. 15 min until stable Regular diet Percocet 2.5 mg. q. 4 hrs p.r.n. for pain Iron supplement q.d. for anemia Discharge to home when stable

LABORATORY REPORTS—PATIENT 7

HEMATOLOGY

DATE: 3/31

Specimen	Results	Normal Values
WBC	7.2	4.3–11.0
RBC	4.0 L	4.5–5.9
HGB	11.0 L	13.5–17.5
HCT	38.0 L	41–52
MCV	94	80–100
MCHC	40	31–57
PLT	300	150–400

Choose the correct principal diagnosis code.

- a. S83.201A
- b. S83.203A
- c. S83.211A
- d. S83.511A
- e. S83.521A

Choose the correct secondary diagnosis code(s).

- a. S83.201A
- b. S83.203A
- c. S83.211A
- d. S83.231A
- e. S83.249A
- f. S83.281A
- g. S83.511A
- h. S83.521A
- i. S83.8X1A
- j. None apply

Practice Case Studies

Choose the correct procedure code(s).

a. 27332-RT
b. 27333
c. 27427-RT, LT
d. 27428
e. 27429-50
f. 29881-RT
g. 29882
h. 29883
i. 29888-RT
j. 29889-50

INPATIENT RECORD—PATIENT 8

DISCHARGE SUMMARY

DATE OF ADMISSION: 1/27   **DATE OF DISCHARGE:** 1/29

DISCHARGE DIAGNOSIS: Congestive heart failure

ADMISSION HISTORY: This is a 57-year-old married white male, referred because of recurrent shortness of breath and cough. He states that he was in his usual state of good health until approximately Christmas, when he developed a persistent cough with associated dyspnea. His dyspnea was most prominent with exertion. He was treated with Ceclor at that time, with some improvement. However, his symptoms recurred and he underwent a second course of antibiotics, again with some improvement. However, his symptoms have now recurred and he is referred for further evaluation.

He has known tricuspid insufficiency, mild left ventricular dysfunction and left ventricular dilation by echocardiogram done 6/2. He had a normal stress ECG 10/3. The patient also has hypertension.

COURSE IN HOSPITAL: The patient was referred because of recurrent shortness of breath and cough. Apparently, the patient had been doing well up until Christmas. His cough was treated with antibiotics with some improvement. His symptoms, however, recurred, requiring a second course of antibiotics.

The patient was admitted with a diagnosis of congestive heart failure. He was started on diuretics with improvement in his physical examination and his symptoms. An echocardiogram was performed, which is described as above.

The patient was extremely anxious to go home and thought that the rest of his care could be accomplished as an outpatient. He is tolerating his medications and will remain on the Capoten and the Lasix and will have a follow-up appointment with his doctor in one to two weeks and I will see him again in approximately 4 weeks. It is recommended at that time that discussion for cardiac catheterization be carried out. This was discussed with the patient during his hospitalization, the reason being that perhaps his tricuspid insufficiency is more significant than what is appreciated on physical examination and by echocardiogram. The catheterization would aid in the evaluation of the etiology of his LV dysfunction and his left ventricular enlargement. He has also been given information about smoking cessation.

INSTRUCTIONS ON DISCHARGE:

1. Capoten 12.5 mg b.i.d.
2. Lasix 40 mg daily
3. Insulin Humulin N 14 in a.m. with 6 of regular and Humulin N 20 units in the p.m. with 12 of regular

Practice Case Studies

HISTORY AND PHYSICAL EXAMINATION—PATIENT 8

ADMITTED: 1/27

REASON FOR ADMISSION: This is a 57-year-old married white male, referred because of recurrent shortness of breath and cough. He states that he was in his usual state of good health until approximately Christmas, when he developed a persistent cough with associated dyspnea. His dyspnea was most prominent with exertion. He was treated with Ceclor at that time with some improvement. However, his symptoms recurred and he underwent a second course of antibiotics, again with some improvement. However, his symptoms have now recurred and he is referred for further evaluation.

He has known moderate tricuspid valve insufficiency, mild left ventricular dysfunction and left ventricular dilation by echocardiogram. He had a normal stress ECG on 10/3.

PAST MEDICAL HISTORY: The patient has a history of type 1 diabetes mellitus. He believes that his most recent cholesterol reading was lower than 200. He previously has been hospitalized for pericarditis and for resection of popliteal artery aneurysm. He has a history of hypertension.

ALLERGIES: None known

CHRONIC MEDICATIONS: Humulin Insulin 6 units of R and 14 units of N in the morning and 12 units of R and 20 units of N in the evening. Lotensin 20 mg PO daily.

He denies any drug allergies.

FAMILY HISTORY: Noncontributory

SOCIAL HISTORY: The patient is married and lives with his wife and smokes one to two packs of cigarettes per day.

REVIEW OF SYSTEMS: Otherwise noncontributory

HISTORY AND PHYSICAL EXAMINATION—PATIENT 8

PHYSICAL EXAMINATION: Reveals a blood pressure of 140/80, pulse 80 and regular. The patient was a pleasant, adult, white male who is in no acute distress. His carotids were without bruits. The jugular venous pulse was normal. Examination of his lungs was remarkable for fine, bibasilar rales. On auscultation of his heart, he has a regular rhythm, a soft murmur consistent with tricuspid insufficiency. Abdominal examination was unremarkable except for the presence of a liver edge just below the costal margin. He had no peripheral edema.

LABORATORY DATA: Thyroid function tests were within normal limits. Total cholesterol level was 194. His HDL and LDL are presently still pending. His blood sugar levels have been well controlled in the low 100s. His electrolytes and SMA 12 are normal as well as his complete blood count.

His EKG on admission revealed sinus rhythm with left atrial enlargement, nonspecific ST-T wave abnormality with poor R wave progression, no acute changes.

His echocardiogram revealed left ventricular enlargement, normal left atrial size at 4 cm, mild overall reduction of left ventricular contractility with diffuse hypokinesis, mild to moderate tricuspid insufficiency.

IMPRESSION:

1. Persistent shortness of breath and cough—possible congestive heart failure; rule out persistent respiratory tract infection
2. Tricuspid insufficiency, left ventricular dysfunction/dilation, by echocardiogram
3. Type 1 diabetes mellitus
4. Smoking history

Practice Case Studies

CONSULTATION—PATIENT 8

DATE: 1/28

Podiatric consultation was requested. The patient's chart was reviewed in the following manner:

H & P, Labs, progress notes, physician's orders, previous consultations and any other pertinent information remaining in the patient's chart.

CHIEF COMPLAINT: Diabetic foot care

PHYSICAL EXAMINATION: The patient is a 57-year-old white male admitted with a history of hypertension and diabetes mellitus, insulin dependent for approximately 7 years. The patient has shortness of breath and is a smoker. The patient states that he has had a problem with one of the valves in his heart for approximately 3 years. The patient had resection of an aneurysm in the right leg in 1989. The patient has no known drug allergies. Bilateral great toenails are hypertrophic and mycotic with in-growing tendencies. The patient has had trauma to both the great toenails at the age of 12 years due to a vehicular accident. Gait analysis will be deferred at this time. Pulses are present in both feet and ankles. The toes are warm. There are no digital lesions at this time. The muscle tone and power are fair. The patient denied having intermittent claudication during gait or phlebitis affecting either lower extremity. The patient does have some numbness of the right great toe, status post-surgery for the popliteal aneurysm.

IMPRESSION:

1. Type 1 diabetes mellitus
2. Congestive heart failure
3. Valvular heart disease
4. Smoker
5. Status post resection of aneurysm of the right leg
6. Hypertension

PLAN: Podiatric consultation; initial; comprehensive. Excisional debridement of hypertrophic mycotic nail plates bilateral great toes—symptomatic

PROCEDURE: Excisional debridement of hypertrophic mycotic nail plates, bilateral great toes, symptomatic

RECOMMENDATIONS: Diabetic foot care q. 1 to 3 months. The patient will be followed p.r.n.

PROGRESS NOTES—PATIENT 8

DATE	NOTE
1/27	Physical examination reveals rales and evidence of valvular heart disease. Will diurese with Lasix and obtain an echocardiogram.
1/28	Patient better today—no shortness of breath, no edema. The importance of smoking cessation was discussed with the patient.
1/29	Will discharge the patient today.

PHYSICIAN'S ORDERS—PATIENT 8

DATE	ORDER
1/27	Chest x-ray
	Monitor input and output
	Lasix 40 mg IV now and 40 mg PO in a.m.
	Schedule patient for an echocardiogram
	CBC
	Consult podiatry for diabetic foot care
	Lotensin 20 mg PO daily in a.m.
1/23	Discharge patient to home.

LABORATORY REPORTS—PATIENT 8

HEMATOLOGY

DATE: 1/27

Specimen	Results	Normal Values
WBC	10	4.3–11.0
RBC	5.0	4.5–5.9
HGB	16.2	13.5–17.5
HCT	48	41–52
MCV	93	80–100
MCHC	35	31–57
PLT	339	150–450

RADIOLOGY REPORT—PATIENT 8

DATE: 1/28

Chest x-ray

DIAGNOSIS: The examination is compared to a prior examination on March 2 of last year. The cardiac silhouette remains at the upper limits of normal in size. The pulmonary vascularity appears slightly congested and there is a right-sided pleural effusion that was not present on the prior examination. There is minimal blunting of the left costophrenic angle. The appearance suggests congestive heart failure.

IMPRESSION: Findings of congestive heart failure

Practice Case Studies

Choose the correct principal diagnosis code.

- a. I10
- b. I11.0
- c. I12.9
- d. I50.9
- e. I50.30

Choose the correct secondary diagnosis code(s).

- a. B35.1
- b. E10.9
- c. E11.9
- d. F17.200
- e. F17.210
- f. I07.1
- g. I50.30
- h. I50.9
- i. L60.2
- j. None apply

Choose the correct procedure code(s).

- a. 0HBQXZZ
- b. 0HBQXZZ
- c. 0HBRXZZ × 2
- d. 0HCQXZZ
- e. 0HCRXZZ
- f. 0HCRXZZ × 2
- g. 0HDQXZZ
- h. 0HDRXZZ
- i. 0HDRXZZ × 2
- j. None apply

Practice Case Studies

EMERGENCY DEPARTMENT RECORD—PATIENT 9

DATE OF ADMISSION: 6/17   **DATE OF DISCHARGE:** 6/17

HISTORY (PROBLEM FOCUSED):

HISTORY OF PRESENT ILLNESS: This 61-year-old Caucasian female who is experiencing dizziness.

PAST MEDICAL HISTORY: The patient has a history of paroxysmal atrial fibrillation well controlled with Coumadin. Also, has type I DM managed with Lantus.

ALLERGIES: None

CHRONIC MEDICATIONS: Coumadin, Lantus insulin

REVIEW OF SYSTEMS: Patient awoke to dizziness today. Upon head movement experiences sensation of vertigo with room spinning. Slight nausea. All other systems reviewed and negative.

PHYSICAL EXAMINATION (PROBLEM FOCUSED):

GENERAL APPEARANCE: This is a well-nourished 61-year-old white female in no apparent distress. HEENT demonstrates dizziness upon movement. Neck veins flat at 40-degree angle. No nodes felt in the neck, carotids, or groin. Carotid pulsations are normal. No bruits heard in the neck. Chest clear on percussion and auscultation. Heart is not enlarged. No thrills or murmurs. Rhythm is regular. BP 127/73. Liver and spleen not palpable. No masses felt in the abdomen. No ascites noted. No edema of the extremities. Pulses in the feet are good.

IMPRESSION: BPPV right ear

PLAN: Zofran for nausea via IV push. CT scan head (results negative)

TREATMENT: Epley maneuver used to address the BPPV

DISCHARGE DIAGNOSIS: BPPV right ear

INSTRUCTIONS ON DISCHARGE: Prescription given for Antivert as directed. Follow up with primary care doctor in 2-3 days.

Emergency Department Evaluation and Management Mapping

The following are the number of acuity points needed to assign a particular level of CPT code:

- Level 1 = 1–20
- Level 2 = 21–35
- Level 3 = 36–47
- Level 4 = 48–60
- Level 5 = > 61
- Critical Care > 61 with constant physician attendance

CPT Codes

- Level 1 = 99281   99281–25 with procedure/laboratory/radiology
- Level 2 = 99282   99282–25 with procedure/laboratory/radiology
- Level 3 = 99283   99283–25 with procedure/laboratory/radiology
- Level 4 = 99284   99284–25 with procedure/laboratory/radiology
- Level 5 = 99285   99285–25 with procedure/laboratory/radiology

Practice Case Studies

Emergency Department Acuity Points					
	5	10	15	20	25
Number of Meds Given	0–2	3–5	6–7	8–9	>10
Extent of Hx	Brief	PF	EPF	Detail	Comprehensive
Extent of Exam	Brief	PF	EPF	Detail	Comprehensive
Number of Tests Ordered	0–1	2–3	4–5	6–7	>8
Number of Supplies Used	1	2–3	4–5	6–7	>8

Choose the correct principal diagnosis code.

- a. H81.10
- b. H81.11
- c. H81.12
- d. H81.13
- e. R42

Choose the correct secondary diagnosis code(s).

- a. E10.9
- b. E11.9
- c. I48.0
- d. I48.2
- e. I48.91
- f. R42
- g. Z79.01
- h. Z79.4
- i. Z79.84
- j. None apply

Choose the correct procedure code(s).

- a. 99282
- b. 99283
- c. 99284
- d. 99285
- e. 99281-25
- f. 99282-25
- g. 99283-25
- h. 99284-25
- i. 99285-25
- j. None apply

CCS

EXAM 1

Exam 1

A blank answer sheet for these multiple-choice questions can be found on page 87.

Domain 1 — Coding Knowledge and Skills

1. The patient is seen in the pain clinic for chronic neoplasm-related pain that was known to be caused by the metastatic bone carcinoma of the vertebra that has spread from carcinoma of the left main bronchus of the lung. How should this be coded?

    a. C34.02, Malignant neoplasm of left main bronchus

    b. G89.3, Neoplasm related pain (acute) (chronic)

    c. G89.3, Neoplasm related pain (acute) (chronic); C79.51, Secondary malignant neoplasm of bone; C34.02, Malignant neoplasm of left main bronchus

    d. C79.51, Secondary malignant neoplasm of bone; G89.3, Neoplasm related pain (acute) (chronic)

2. A child is seen in the emergency department for second- and third-degree burns of the left lower leg and second- and third-degree burns of the lower back, for a total of 16 percent of body surface area burned, 9 percent of which are third-degree burns. What is the correct code assignment?

    a. T24.301A, T21.34XA, T31.10

    b. T24.302D, T21.34XD, T31.10

    c. T24.302A, T21.34XA, T31.10

    d. T24.301D, T21.34XD, T31.10

3. A patient underwent excision of a malignant lesion of the skin of the chest that measured 1.0 cm, and there was a 0.2-cm margin on both sides. Based on the 2020 CPT codes, which code would be used for the procedure?

    a. 11401, Excision, benign lesion including margins, except skin tag (unless listed elsewhere), trunk, arms or legs; excised diameter 0.6 to 1.0 cm

    b. 11601, Excision, malignant lesion including margins, trunk, arms, or legs; excised diameter 0.6 to 1.0 cm

    c. 11602, Excision, malignant lesion including margins, trunk, arms, or legs; excised diameter 1.1 to 2.0 cm

    d. 11402, Excision, benign lesion including margins, except skin tag (unless listed elsewhere), trunk, arms or legs; excised diameter 1.1 to 2.0 cm

4. A laparoscopic tubal ligation with Falope ring is completed. What is the correct CPT code assignment?

49321	Laparoscopy, surgical; with biopsy (single or multiple)
58662	Laparoscopy, surgical; with fulguration or excision of lesions of the ovary, pelvic viscera, or peritoneal surface by any method
58670	Laparoscopy, surgical; with fulguration of oviducts (with or without transection)
58671	Laparoscopy, surgical; with occlusion of oviducts by device (eg, band, clip, or Falope ring)

    a. 58662

    b. 58670

    c. 58671

    d. 49321

5. A patient is admitted to the hospital for pain due to displacement of pacemaker electrode. The patient also has hypothyroidism due to partial thyroidectomy seven years ago and a breast cyst. Using a guide wire, the pacemaker electrode was relocated and Synthroid was given during hospitalization. The codes (excluding External Cause codes) that should be assigned are:

T82.110A	Breakdown (mechanical) of cardiac electrode, initial encounter
T82.110D	Breakdown (mechanical) of cardiac electrode, subsequent encounter
T82.120A	Displacement of cardiac electrode, initial encounter
T82.120S	Displacement of cardiac electrode, sequela
N60.09	Solitary cyst of unspecified breast
E89.0	Postsurgical hypothyroidism
02WA3MZ	Revision of cardiac lead in heart, percutaneous approach
02WA4MZ	Revision of cardiac lead in heart, percutaneous endoscopic approach
02WA0MZ	Revision of cardiac lead in heart, open approach

a. T82.110A, E89.0, 02WA3MZ

b. T82.110D, E89.0, N60.09, 02WA4MZ

c. T82.120A, E89.0, 02WA3MZ

d. T82.120S, E89.0, N60.09, 02WA0MZ

6. A maternity patient is admitted in labor at 43 weeks. She has a spontaneous delivery with vacuum extraction to facilitate the baby's delivery. Which of the following would be the principal diagnosis?

O80	Encounter for full-term uncomplicated delivery
O48.0	Post-term pregnancy
O48.1	Prolonged pregnancy
O66.5	Attempted application of vacuum extractor and forceps

a. O48.0

b. O48.1

c. O80

d. O66.5

7. A patient is admitted to the hospital due to a fracture of the right hip and is scheduled for an open reduction with internal fixation. The patient developed cardiac arrhythmia which results in an inability to do the planned surgery. What is the principal diagnosis?

a. Status post fracture

b. Cardiac arrhythmia

c. Right hip fracture

d. Cancelled procedure

8. A 45-year-old man with known AIDS is admitted to the hospital for treatment of HIV-related *Pneumocystis carinii* pneumonia. What is the principal diagnosis code?

a. B20

b. J18.9

c. B59

d. Any of the above

9. Patient admitted with hemorrhage due to placenta previa with twin pregnancy. This patient had two prior (cesarean section) deliveries. Emergency C-section was performed due to the hemorrhage. The appropriate principal diagnosis would be:

   a. Prior cesarean sections
   b. Placenta previa without hemorrhage
   c. Twin gestation
   d. Placenta previa with hemorrhage

10. A patient presents to a facility with a history of prostate cancer and mental confusion on admission. The patient completed radiation therapy for prostatic carcinoma three years ago and is status post a radical resection of the prostate. A CT scan of the brain reveals metastatic carcinoma of the brain. The correct coding and sequencing of this patient's record is:

    a. Metastatic carcinoma of the brain, carcinoma of the prostate, mental confusion
    b. Mental confusion, history of carcinoma of the prostate, metastatic carcinoma of the brain
    c. Metastatic carcinoma of the brain, history of carcinoma of the prostate
    d. Carcinoma of the prostate, metastatic carcinoma to the brain

11. A patient with GERD presents to a facility for upper endoscopy submucosal injection of material near the lower esophageal sphincter. The correct coding and sequencing of this patient's record is:

Code	Description
K20.9	Esophagitis, unspecified
K21.0	Gastro-esophageal disease with esophagitis
K21.9	Gastro-esophageal disease without esophagitis
43235	Esophagogastroduodenoscopy, flexible, transoral; diagnostic, including collection of specimen(s) by brushing or washing, when performed (separate procedure)
43236	with directed submucosal injection(s), any substance
43257	with delivery of thermal energy to the muscle of lower esophageal sphincter and/or gastric cardia, for treatment of gastroesophageal reflux disease
43270	with ablation of tumor(s), polyp(s), or other lesion(s) (includes pre- and post- dilation and guide wire passage, when performed.
–58	Staged or related procedure or service by the same physician or other qualified health care professional during the postoperative period
–59	Distinct procedural service

    a. K20.9, 43257
    b. K21.0, 43235, 43236
    c. K21.9, 43236
    d. K21.9, K20.9, 43270–58, 43236–59

12. According to CPT, an endoscopy that is undertaken to the level of the midtransverse colon would be coded as a:

    a. Proctosigmoidoscopy
    b. Sigmoidoscopy
    c. Colonoscopy
    d. Proctoscopy

13. If a patient is admitted with pneumococcal pneumonia and severe pneumococcal sepsis, the coder should:

    a. Assign codes for sepsis and pneumonia
    b. Assign codes for sepsis, pneumonia, and severe sepsis
    c. Assign only a code for pneumococcal pneumonia
    d. Review the chart to determine if septic shock could be coded first

14. A female patient with terminal carcinoma of the breast, metastatic to the liver, brain, and intrahepatic and extrahepatic bile ducts, was admitted with dehydration. Patient was rehydrated with IVs and discharged, with no treatment given to the cancer. What are the codes assigned?

    a. E86.0, C50.919, C78.7, C79.31, C78.89
    b. C50.919, E86.0, C78.7, C79.31
    c. C50.919, E86.9, C78.7, C79.31
    d. E86.9, C50.919, C78.7, C79.31, C78.89

15. 45-year-old patient admitted with insulin dependent diabetes. The type of diabetes is not specified in the medical record. How should this be coded?

    a. E11.9, Z79.4
    b. E11.8, Z79.4
    c. Z79.4, E11.8
    d. Query the provider for the type of diabetes

16. A patient was admitted to the hospital with unstable angina and congestive heart failure. The unstable angina is treated with nitrates, and intravenous Lasix is given to manage the heart failure. What is the appropriate coding action?

    a. Assign only the code for the congestive heart failure.
    b. Assign the codes for the unstable angina and congestive heart failure, sequence either first.
    c. Query the physician about which diagnoses to code.
    d. Assign only the code for the unstable angina.

17. A patient presents to the outpatient surgical area for a cystoscopy with multiple biopsies of the bladder. The patient's presenting symptom is hematuria. What is the correct facility code assignment for this procedure?

    | 52000 | Cystourethroscopy (separate procedure) |
    | 52204 | Cystourethroscopy with biopsy(s) |
    | −22 | Increased procedural services |

    a. 52000
    b. 52000-22
    c. 52204
    d. 52204, 52204-22

18. A patient has blepharoplasty of the left upper eyelid. What modifier should be used with the procedure?

    a. LT

    b. TA

    c. E1

    d. F2

19. Facilities may use X modifiers in place of which other modifier?

    a. 25

    b. 27

    c. 52

    d. 59

20. A sigmoidectomy takes the physician more time than originally planned. The reason was extensive lysis of adhesions which took over two hours. What modifier can the physician use to indicate this procedure required increased time?

    a. 22

    b. 26

    c. 52

    d. 59

21. A patient is admitted to the hospital with shortness of breath and congestive heart failure and subsequently develops respiratory failure. The patient undergoes intubation with ventilator management. The correct sequencing of the diagnoses in this case would be:

    a. Congestive heart failure and respiratory failure

    b. Respiratory failure

    c. Respiratory failure and congestive heart failure

    d. Shortness of breath, congestive heart failure, and respiratory failure

22. A patient was admitted with end stage renal disease (ESRD) following kidney transplant. The patient undergoes dialysis during admission. The patient's angina and chronic obstructive pulmonary disease are managed with medication while admitted. The diagnoses would be sequenced as:

    a. Status post kidney transplant; ESRD, chronic obstructive pulmonary disease; angina

    b. ESRD; status post kidney transplant; chronic obstructive pulmonary disease; angina

    c. Angina; ESRD, status post kidney transplant; chronic obstructive pulmonary disease

    d. Chronic obstructive pulmonary disease; ESRD; status post kidney transplant; angina

23. This patient was admitted for chemotherapy due to a primary hepatocellular carcinoma of the transplanted liver. What codes are assigned?

    a. C80.2, T86.49, Z51.11, C22.0

    b. C22.0, C80.2, Z51.11, T86.49

    c. Z51.11, T86.49, C80.2, C22.0

    d. T86.49, C80.2, C22.0, Z51.11

24. A patient comes to the ER with chest pain and shortness of breath. An EKG was performed, and the patient's history of COPD was noted. Unstable angina was diagnosed as the chest pain came on while the patient was at rest and did not resolve with nitroglycerin. The patient was admitted for a left heart catheterization, coronary arteriography using two catheters and left ventricular angiography. The patient was found to have arteriosclerotic heart disease. The patient has no history of cardiac surgery. The appropriate sequencing of ICD-10-CM and CPT codes would be:

I20.0	Unstable angina
I20.9	Angina pectoris, unspecified
I25.10	Atherosclerotic heart disease of native coronary artery without angina pectoris
I25.110	Atherosclerotic heart disease of native coronary artery with unstable angina pectoris
I25.119	Atherosclerotic heart disease of native coronary artery with unspecified angina pectoris
J44.9	Chronic obstructive pulmonary disease
R06.02	Shortness of breath
R07.9	Chest pain, unspecified
93452	Left heart catheterization including intraprocedural injection(s) for left ventriculography, imaging supervision and interpretation, when performed
93453	Combined right and left heart catheterization including intraprocedural injection(s) for left ventriculography, imaging supervision and interpretation, when performed
93454	Catheter placement in coronary artery(s) for coronary angiography, including intraprocedural injection(s) for coronary angiography, imaging supervision and interpretation;
93458	with left heart catheterization including intraprocedural injection(s) for left ventriculography, when performed

   a. R07.9, R06.02, I25.119, 93452, 93458
   b. J44.9, I20.0, I25.110, 93454, 93453
   c. I20.9, J44.9, 93453
   d. I25.110, J44.9, 93458

25. An obstetric patient is admitted with vaginal spotting and fever. She is found to have been treated for a miscarriage (spontaneous abortion), which was resolved two weeks prior to this admission. She is treated with aspiration dilation and curettage and products of conception are found. She is found to be septic. Which of the following is the correct sequencing of the diagnoses for this case?

   a. A41.9, O03.37
   b. O26.859, R51
   c. R51, O26.859
   d. O03.37, A41.9

26. Patient was admitted with pneumonia. Sputum cultures on day three of admission indicate a *Klebsiella* pneumonia. What is the POA status for the *Klebsiella* pneumonia and why?

   a. Y, because the pneumonia was present on admission, even though the organism was not verified until days later
   b. N, because the type of pneumonia was not verified until after admission
   c. U, because the coder must query the physician for POA status in this case
   d. W, because the physician cannot tell if the reason for the pneumonia at the time of admission was the *Klebsiella* or not

27. A patient has a hernia repair done as an outpatient. In recovery, the patient develops tachycardia and shortness of breath, is diagnosed with postoperative atrial fibrillation, and is subsequently admitted. What is the POA indicator for the postoperative atrial fibrillation?

   a. Y
   b. N
   c. U
   d. W

28. A patient is admitted with acute gastritis. On the second day of admission, the patient has hematemesis. The patient is also being treated for long-standing hypertension and diabetes, along with recently diagnosed hypothyroidism. Which of the patient's diagnoses will have a POA indicator of N?

   a. Diabetes
   b. Hypothyroidism
   c. Hypertension
   d. Acute gastritis

29. Which type of conditions are always considered present on admission?

   a. Obstetrical
   b. Congenital
   c. Those with an acute exacerbation
   d. Those that represent an injury

30. A patient is admitted for seizures. What is the appropriate POA for the external cause code of W06.XXXA assigned because the patient fell out of bed during a seizure in the emergency department?

   a. Y
   b. N
   c. U
   d. W

31. The outpatient code editor (OCE) has all of the following types of edits *except*:

   a. Sex and procedure edits
   b. Valid diagnosis code edits
   c. Invalid revenue code edits
   d. Diagnosis and age edits

32. Determining medical necessity for outpatient services includes all the following *except*:

   a. Local coverage determinations (LCDs)
   b. National coverage determinations (NCDs)
   c. Diagnoses linked to procedures by claims-processing software tests ensuring that the procedure is cross-referenced, or linked, correctly to an acceptable diagnosis code for that service
   d. Requiring new HCPCS codes be developed to replace codes in the CPT code book

33. The National Correct Coding Initiative (NCCI) Edits apply to services billed by:

    a. The same provider, for same beneficiary, on same date of service
    b. All providers, for the same beneficiary, on the same date of service
    c. The same provider, for the same beneficiary, for all dates of service related to the encounter
    d. All providers, for the same beneficiary, for all dates of service related to the encounter

34. If the principal diagnosis is an initial anterior wall myocardial infarction, which procedure will result in the highest MS-DRG assignment?

    a. Mechanical ventilator
    b. Insertion central venous catheter
    c. Right heart cardiac catheterization
    d. Transbronchial lung biopsy

35. Medicare payment to physicians for services rendered is made under the:

    a. Outpatient Prospective Payment System
    b. Resource-based Relative Value Scale
    c. Ambulatory Payment Classification
    d. Conditions of Participation

36. Inpatient procedures are coded with:

    a. HCPCS
    b. CPT
    c. ICD-10-PCS
    d. ICD-O

37. Under the Inpatient Prospective Payment System (IPPS), what can be used to measure the cost of care for inpatients?

    a. MS-DRG assignment
    b. RBRVS
    c. Case-mix index
    d. SOI-ROM

38. The abstracting of this data element has an impact on the DRG reimbursement.

    a. Date of service
    b. Discharge disposition
    c. Admission source
    d. Medical record number

39. Which of the following is a data element that coders typically are tasked with abstracting?

    a. Blood type
    b. Date of admission
    c. Sex
    d. Date of surgery

40. Dr. Jones is the attending physician for a patient admitted with aspiration of a ballpoint pen cap. Dr. Westwood is the provider who performed a direct laryngoscopy with foreign body removal on the patient the afternoon of admission. Monitoring of the patient's respiratory status continued for 36 hours after the procedure as severe swelling of the larynx was noted during the laryngoscopy. On the morning of discharge, the patient was noted to have acute, suppurative otitis media of the right ear and Dr. Phillips performed a myringotomy with tube insertion under general anesthesia with assistance from Dr. Johannsen, the resident.

    Upon discharge, which physician will be assigned to the principal procedure that was performed?

    a. Dr. Jones

    b. Dr. Westwood

    c. Dr. Johannsen

    d. Dr. Phillips

41. When a patient goes home with an order for home health to start one week after an inpatient admission, this is categorized as a(n):

    a. Discharge

    b. Transfer

    c. Readmission

    d. Outlier

42. A patient is admitted with an acute inferior myocardial infarction and discharged alive. Which condition would increase the MS-DRG weight?

    a. Respiratory failure

    b. Atrial fibrillation

    c. Hypertension

    d. History of myocardial infarction

43. Documentation in the record reveals that a patient is admitted with an acute exacerbation of COPD (MS-DRG 192). A higher-paying MS-DRG may be appropriate if documentation is present in the record at the time the decision was made to admit the patient that confirms a diagnosis associated with which of the following?

    a. Angina and treated with nitroglycerin prn

    b. Atrial fibrillation and underwent a cardioversion

    c. Respiratory failure treated with intubation and mechanical ventilation for 23 hours

    d. Anemia and was given a blood transfusion

44. A female patient is diagnosed with congestive heart failure. Which of the following will increase the MS-DRG weight if present on admission?

    a. Atrial fibrillation

    b. Stage III pressure ulcer of coccyx

    c. Blood loss anemia

    d. Coronary artery disease

45. Major complications and comorbidities (MCCs) are determined to require the greatest degree of resources with a payment group and also reflect the greatest _____.

    a. ROM
    b. ROI
    c. SOI
    d. SNF

46. Which of the following diagnoses qualifies as MCC?

    a. Coronary artery disease
    b. Aortic stenosis
    c. Type 2 myocardial infarction
    d. Unspecified atrial fibrillation

Domain 2 Coding Documentation

47. A 7-year-old patient was admitted to the emergency department for treatment of shortness of breath. The patient is given epinephrine and nebulizer treatments. The shortness of breath and wheezing are unabated following treatment. What diagnosis should be suspected?

    a. Acute bronchitis
    b. Acute bronchitis with chronic obstructive pulmonary disease
    c. Asthma with status asthmaticus
    d. Chronic obstructive asthma

48. A 23-year-old female is admitted for shock following treatment of an ectopic pregnancy. This encounter would be coded as:

    a. O03.81, Spontaneous abortion complicated by shock
    b. O08.3, Complication following ectopic and molar pregnancies
    c. R57.9, Shock NOS
    d. T81.10XA, Postoperative shock

49. A patient is discharged with a diagnosis of acute pulmonary edema due to congestive heart failure. What condition(s) should be coded?

    a. Acute pulmonary edema
    b. Congestive heart failure
    c. Acute pulmonary edema and congestive heart failure
    d. Unable to determine based on the information provided

50. A 65-year-old male patient is being assessed for possible colon cancer and treated in the special procedure unit of the hospital. He undergoes a colonoscopy with biopsy of a suspicious area in the transverse colon using the cold biopsy forceps. In addition, a colonic ultrasound is performed, with transmural biopsy of an area of the mesentery adjacent to the transverse colon. Assign the appropriate CPT codes.

    a. 45384, 45342

    b. 45380, 45391

    c. 45384, 45392

    d. 45380, 45392

51. FNA and core biopsies are done on the same breast lesion, in the same session, on the same day, both performed with fluoroscopic guidance. What codes would be assigned?

    a. 19100, 10007-59

    b. 10007 ×2, 19100 ×2, 77002

    c. 10007, 10008, 19100 ×2

    d. 19100, 10007-59, 77002

52. The physician removes all of a right thyroid lobe without isthmusectomy. The physician exposes the thyroid via a transverse cervical incision in the skin line. The platysmas are divided and the strap muscles separated in the midline. The thyroid lobe to be excised is isolated and superior and inferior thyroid vessels serving that lobe are ligated. Parathyroid glands are preserved. The thyroid gland is divided in the midline of the isthmus over the anterior trachea. The thyroid lobe is resected. The platysmas and skin are closed. What code should be assigned?

    a. 0GTH4ZZ

    b. 0GTL0ZZ

    c. 0GTH0ZZ

    d. 0GTL4ZZ

53. The physician inserts a speculum into the vagina to view the cervix. The cervix was dilated. The endometrial lining of the uterus is scraped on all sides for therapeutic purposes. What code should be assigned?

    a. 0UDB7ZX

    b. 0UDB7ZZ

    c. 0UDB8ZZ

    d. 0U5B7ZZ

54. A 28-year-old male with a history of IV heroin dependence is admitted for pneumonia. A pulmonologist is consulted to assist with the patient's treatment and an antibiotic for *Pneumocystis carinii* pneumonia is administered. Low potassium is treated as well. The final diagnoses were coded as: B20, B59, E87.6, and F11.21. What is the discrepancy noted between the coding and the documentation?

    a. The "history of" code reflects abuse rather than dependence

    b. The correct code for the pneumonia should be J18.9

    c. The assignment of B20 has no supportive documentation

    d. The hypokalemia should not be coded as that is integral to the pneumonia

55. A patient is admitted post–back surgery with uncontrolled pain and leakage at the surgical site. Vitals show a fever of 101 with some tachycardia noted as well. The attending physician documents inflammation, with an infectious disease consultant documenting *Staphylococcus aureus* infection based on the lab culture. How should the coder resolve the discrepancy between the diagnoses documented?

    a. Code the inflammation since that is what the attending physician documented
    b. Code the infection since the consultant was specific regarding the type of infection
    c. Code the infection based on the lab culture results
    d. Query the attending physician to clarify the conflicting documentation

56. A coder has noted that a particular nurse practitioner is sending orders for outpatient testing with the diagnosis listed as "possible" or "rule out" without any accompanying signs or symptoms or abnormal findings suggestive of the possible diagnosis. What action should the coder take?

    a. Nothing, code the diagnosis as if it exists since this is an outpatient
    b. Use an observation code for the encounter
    c. Ask for outpatient CDI specialist to educate the NP on the guidelines for outpatient coding which do not permit the use of "possible" or "rule out" diagnoses
    d. Report the nurse practitioner to quality management and billing as this practice is causing billing delays and increase in the discharge not final billed metric

57. An operative report indicates the physician performed metatarsal surgery but all other information in the record points to need for metacarpal surgery. What step should the coder take upon this discovery?

    a. Code the metatarsal surgery as that is what is documented in the operative report
    b. Code the metacarpal surgery since the op report was clearly an error
    c. Query the physician to determine which body area the surgery involved
    d. Suspend the chart and contact the coding supervisor as to which procedure to code

58. A patient is seen in the ED with leg edema and headache. The patient denies shortness of breath, chest pain, and chills. The patient has a chest x-ray, CT of the head, and lab work. A doppler scan was done to evaluate for a DVT, which was negative. Final diagnoses in the ED was swelling of leg, migraine, and chest pain. What is the discrepancy in this documentation?

    a. Swelling is not documented outside the final diagnosis
    b. There was no chest pain by patient report
    c. Possible DVT should have been listed as final diagnosis
    d. No testing was provided to assess migraine

Domain 3 Provider Queries

59. The most challenging type of provider query is issued for:

    a. Determining cause and effect
    b. Establishing clinical validation
    c. Resolving documentation conflict
    d. Clarifying acuity or specificity

60. When creating a compliant query to clarify conflicting information from the surgeon and the attending physician, to whom should the query be directed?

   a. Surgeon
   b. Attending physician
   c. Medical staff director
   d. Medical records committee chairperson

61. When a compliant query remains unanswered, what is the next step for the coder?

   a. Ask the HIM director to place the physician on suspension until the query is answered.
   b. Alert the CEO that the query is outstanding, requesting a fine until the query is answered.
   c. Refer to the internal escalation policy and follow the process outlined therein.
   d. Report the physician to the peer review committee for disciplinary measures.

62. When creating compliant queries coders should:

   a. Query once without further follow up
   b. Query multiple times until the desired diagnosis is provided
   c. Query once with additional follow up if necessary
   d. Query unlimited times until every discrepancy is resolved

63. Verbal queries:

   a. Are not permissible in any circumstance
   b. Must have a written response in the record for coding purposes
   c. Have different rules or criteria than written queries
   d. Are not required to be documented as long as the physician responds verbally

64. A patient is admitted with a high temperature, lethargy, hypotension, tachycardia, oliguria, and elevated WBC. The patient also has more than 100,000 organisms of *Escherichia coli* per cc of urine. The attending physician documents "urosepsis." What is the next step for the coder?

   a. Code sepsis as the principal with a secondary diagnosis of urinary tract infection due to *E. coli*.
   b. Code urinary tract infection with sepsis as a secondary diagnosis.
   c. Query the physician to determine if the patient is being treated for sepsis, highlighting the clinical signs and symptoms.
   d. Ask the physician whether the patient had septic shock so that this may be used as the principal diagnosis.

65. A patient has findings suggestive of chronic obstructive pulmonary disease (COPD) on chest x-ray. The attending physician mentions the x-ray finding in one progress note but no medication, treatment, or further evaluation is provided. The coder should:

   a. Query the attending physician regarding the x-ray finding
   b. Code the condition because the documentation reflects it
   c. Question the radiologist regarding whether to code this condition
   d. Use a code from abnormal findings to reflect the condition

66. If a patient undergoes an inpatient procedure and the final summary diagnosis is different from the diagnosis on the pathology report, the coder should:

    a. Code only from the discharge diagnoses

    b. Code the diagnosis reflected on the pathology report

    c. Code the most severe symptom

    d. Query the attending physician as to the final diagnosis

67. A 56-year-old woman is admitted to an acute-care facility from a skilled nursing facility. The patient has multiple sclerosis and hypertension. During the course of hospitalization, a decubitus ulcer is found and debrided at the bedside by a physician. There is no typed operative report and no pathology report. The coder should:

    a. Use an excisional debridement code as these charts are rarely reviewed to verify the excisional debridement.

    b. Code with a nonexcisional debridement procedure code.

    c. Query the healthcare provider who performed the procedure to determine if the debridement was excisional.

    d. Eliminate the procedure code all together.

68. Patient presents with lower left quadrant abdominal pain with normal white cell count. X-ray showed sigmoid diverticulitis. Patient underwent a resection of sigmoid colon with anastomosis, developing a postoperative ileus after surgery. Nausea abated after resolution of the ileus. What is the query opportunity for this case?

    a. Was the diverticulitis perforated?

    b. Was the nausea postoperative?

    c. Was there an associated abscess with the diverticulitis?

    d. Was the postoperative ileus a complication?

69. A 64-year-old female is admitted to the hospital with nausea, vomiting, and edema. The patient has a history of diabetes and takes Metformin and Lisinopril as prescribed. Blood sugar and blood pressure are monitored while admitted. On the discharge summary, the final diagnoses of acute renal failure and diabetes are documented. What is the query opportunity for this record?

    a. Is the acute renal failure linked to the diabetes?

    b. Does the patient have hypertension?

    c. Does the patient have chronic renal failure?

    d. Is the diabetes out of control?

Domain 4 Regulatory Compliance

70. Most hospitals require a medical record to be completed within:

    a. 5 days

    b. 10 days

    c. 7 days

    d. 30 days

71. To correct an entry in a paper-based medical record, the provider should:

a. Draw a single line through the error, add a note explaining the error, initial and date, add the correct information in chronological order

b. Draw a double line through the error, initial and date, add the reason for the correction

c. Draw a single line through the error, and add the correct information in chronological order

d. Draw several lines through the error, obliterate the documentation as much as possible, initial and date, add the correct information in chronological order

72. After a patient is discharged from the hospital, the medical record must be reviewed for:

a. Inclusion of all incident reports

b. Certain basic reports (for example, history and physical, discharge summary, etc.)

c. Voided prescription pads

d. Personal case notes from all mental health providers

73. A completed and signed operative report needs clarification of the size of the skin lesions that were removed. What process is used for that clarification?

a. Amendment

b. Addendum

c. Update

d. Revision

Use the information in the following table to answer questions 74 through 76.

Billing Number	Status Indicator*	CPT/HCPCS	APC
989323	V	99285–25	05025
989323	T	25500	05111
989323	X	72050	05522
989323	S	72128	05522
989323	N	70450	05522

*Status Indicators.

N—No additional payment, payment included in line items with APCs for incidental service
S— Significant Procedure, Not Discounted when Multiple
T—Significant Procedure, Multiple Reduction Applies
V—Medical visit to clinic or emergency department
X—Ancillary Services

74. The information in the table represents all the CPT/HCPCS codes and associated information pertinent to a patient's encounter for care. From the information provided, how many APCs would impact this patient's total reimbursement?

a. 1

b. 5

c. 4

d. Unable to determine

75. What percentage will the facility be paid for procedure code 25500?

    a. 50%
    b. 75%
    c. 0%
    d. 100%

76. If another status T procedure were performed, how much would the facility receive for the second status T procedure?

    a. 50%
    b. 75%
    c. 0%
    d. 100%

77. Which of the following would be considered a hospital-acquired condition when the POA indicator is N?

    a. DVT following a gastric procedure
    b. Diabetes with neuropathy
    c. Catheter-associated urinary tract infection
    d. Foreign body in the thumb

78. A patient is admitted with abdominal pain and is found to have a perforation due to large intestine diverticulitis. A colectomy is performed. Following the procedure, there is a slight fever, and elevated white count. An x-ray shows a metallic object in the area of the previous surgery. A return to the OR with reopening of the wound shows that a piece of a surgical blade had broken off and been left in the wound. Which of the following diagnoses is a hospital acquired condition and will bear the POA indicator of N?

    a. R50.9
    b. K57.20
    c. D72.829
    d. T81.520A

79. When a POA indicator for a HAC that is the only CC/MCC condition on the record is listed as N, what happens to the reimbursement for that account?

    a. Nothing, the reimbursement is not impacted as this is an internal quality monitoring code
    b. The reimbursement goes up since the condition was not present on admission and more resources were needed to care for the patient
    c. The reimbursement goes down since the condition was not present on admission and could/should have been prevented using best practices
    d. The reimbursement is placed on hold until the physician clarifies why the patient did not have the condition on admission

80. Which of the following may be considered a hospital-acquired condition?

    a. Diabetic foot ulcer
    b. Stage 2 coccyx pressure ulcer
    c. Calf ulcer, left leg, with muscle necrosis
    d. Right elbow pressure ulcer, stage 4

81. Which of the following statements best describes how the retention of records should be determined?

    a. Unless state law requires longer periods of time, specific patient health information should be retained for HIPAA established minimum time periods.
    b. AHIMA has published specific guidelines for retention of health information and these guidelines should be followed for records retention.
    c. The Joint Commission has developed standards for retention of health information which must be followed to maintain accreditation and these standards should be adhered to with regard to time frames.
    d. Health records should be retained according to their use in a facility and the state and federal laws do not apply to the retention of this health information.

82. The form that must be completed in order to permit a specific disclosure of protected health information is called a(n):

    a. Authorization
    b. Consent
    c. Access
    d. Redisclosure

83. The minimum necessary requirement would apply in which scenario below?

    a. When disclosure is to the secretary of HHS for investigation
    b. When disclosure is required by law
    c. When disclosure is for payment
    d. When disclosure is made to the personal representative of the individual

84. What is the term used when protected health information has been disclosed inappropriately?

    a. Exposure
    b. Breach
    c. Violation
    d. Infraction

85. What is the term used for applying the HIPAA privacy rule over state rule(s) which are less strict?

    a. Exception
    b. Preemption
    c. Exclusion
    d. Predominance

86. A contract coder works for a hospital and, in the course of daily work, routinely accesses protected patient health information. Under HIPAA, what should be in place to permit access and protect patient privacy?

    a. AHIMA credential
    b. Business associate agreement
    c. Vendor license
    d. Patient authorization

87. Based on the AHIMA Code of Ethics, which of the following is *not* considered an ethical activity?

    a. Coding audits

    b. Using medical records for educational purposes within the department

    c. Reviewing the history and physical of a coworker when not part of work assignment

    d. Completion of code assignment

88. After consulting with a physician, a coding supervisor has issued an internal policy stating that all bedside debridement be coded as excisional. Is this an ethical practice for a coder to follow? Why or why not?

    a. Yes, physician guidance provided basis for the policy.

    b. Yes, coders must follow internal policies of the facilities where they are employed.

    c. No, coding supervisors cannot make internal policies without approval of administration.

    d. No, internal policies cannot conflict with requirements provided in coding guidelines, conventions, and so on.

89. It is unethical for a coder to query:

    a. Retrospectively

    b. When the response will impact reimbursement

    c. Based on information in a previous encounter

    d. Multiple times on the same patient record

90. A patient came in for surgery and developed a post-operative infection. The patient had multiple comorbid conditions, which provided several CC and MCC conditions that were captured in coding. However, the coder left off the post-op infection code knowing it would impact the physician's quality of care score. Is this acceptable, ethical practice? Why or why not?

    a. Yes; since it will not impact reimbursement, there is no issue.

    b. Yes; coders have discretion in which codes to assign on every case.

    c. No; the coding of the post-op infection would have impacted reimbursement.

    d. No; coders cannot intentionally omit codes in order to affect quality scores.

91. Which of the following is an ethical way to handle an internal coding policy that conflicts with coding guidelines?

    a. Report the concern through the organization's compliance hotline

    b. Talk with fellow coders to develop your own plan

    c. Ignore the internal policy and follow coding guidelines

    d. Wait six months to see if the policy gets changed and then report your concern

92. In addition to credentialed coders, AHIMA's Standards of Ethical Coding apply to which groups below?

    a. Non-credentialed coders and students

    b. Students and attorneys

    c. Attorneys and auditors

    d. Case managers and non-credentialed coders

93. A diabetic patient was admitted for a treatment of a pressure ulcer. The patient also has a history of diabetic neuropathy and retinopathy. The patient is blind and additional nursing care and extended time with the patient was required. Which conditions should be coded at discharge?

    a. Pressure ulcer, history of neurologic condition, history of retinal condition, diabetes
    b. Pressure ulcer, diabetic neuropathy and diabetic retinopathy, and blindness
    c. Pressure ulcer, diabetic neuropathy
    d. Pressure ulcer, diabetic retinopathy, and blindness

94. A patient admitted with shoulder pain has an inpatient discharge with principal diagnosis of either peptic ulcer or cholecystitis documented on the history and physical. Both are equally treated and well documented. A coder should:

    a. Code based on the circumstances of admission and if both are equally treated, code either as principal
    b. Use a code from the abnormal findings category
    c. Code to the most severe symptom only
    d. Code shoulder pain followed by both peptic ulcer, cholecystitis

95. During an admission for congestive heart failure (CHF), a chest x-ray was done to evaluate the severity of the CHF. An asymptomatic hernia was also found for which *no* treatment or evaluation was done. What is the reason that the hernia should not be coded?

    a. The patient's primary condition of interest is the CHF.
    b. The hernia is an incidental finding and does not meet the UHDDS requirements.
    c. The patient is asymptomatic.
    d. The condition does not impact the reimbursement.

96. According to the UHDDS, section III, the definition of *other diagnoses* is all conditions that:

    a. Coexist at the time of admission, that develop subsequently, or that affect the treatment received or the length of stay
    b. Receive evaluation and are documented by the physician
    c. Receive clinical evaluation, therapeutic treatment, further evaluation, extend the length of stay, increase nursing monitoring/care
    d. Are considered to be essential by the physicians involved and are reflected in the record

97. Which patient specific UHDDS items also have the potential to an impact on MS-DRG assignment?

    a. Race and residence
    b. Residence and sex
    c. Sex and discharge disposition
    d. Discharge disposition and race

Multiple Choice Exam 1 Answers

1.	26.	51.	76.
2.	27.	52.	77.
3.	28.	53.	78.
4.	29.	54.	79.
5.	30.	55.	80.
6.	31.	56.	81.
7.	32.	57.	82.
8.	33.	58.	83.
9.	34.	59.	84.
10.	35.	60.	85.
11.	36.	61.	86.
12.	37.	62.	87.
13.	38.	63.	88.
14.	39.	64.	89.
15.	40.	65.	90.
16.	41.	66.	91.
17.	42.	67.	92.
18.	43.	68.	93.
19.	44.	69.	94.
20.	45.	70.	95.
21.	46.	71.	96.
22.	47.	72.	97.
23.	48.	73.	
24.	49.	74.	
25.	50.	75.	

EXAM 1
CASE STUDIES

CCS

SAME DAY SURGERY SUMMARY—PATIENT 1

HISTORY AND PHYSICAL EXAMINATION

REASON FOR ADMISSION: Breast mass

HISTORY OF PRESENT ILLNESS: The patient is a 57-year-old woman who had a routine mammogram performed last week. A lump was noted in the upper, outer quadrant of the right breast, about 1.2 cm in size. The patient was referred to me. After an explanation to the patient about the condition, a needle localization breast biopsy was performed which revealed intraductal carcinoma in situ.

PAST MEDICAL HISTORY: Noncontributory

ALLERGIES: None known

CHRONIC MEDICATIONS: None

SOCIAL HISTORY: The patient is a 57-year-old female who is married and lives with her husband. She is a nondrinker and a nonsmoker.

REVIEW OF SYSTEMS: The patient has normal bowels. There is no hematuria or dysuria. The patient has had two colds in the past 6 weeks. She states that she has been having some difficulty sleeping because of worry over this breast mass.

PHYSICAL EXAMINATION: This is a well-developed, well-nourished 57-year-old female who appears younger than her stated age.

    HEENT: PERRLA with supple neck

    LUNGS: The lungs are clear to percussion and auscultation.

    CHEST: The heart has normal rhythm and pulse. There is a mass in the right breast.

    ABDOMEN: Abdomen reveals no masses; bowel sounds are heard.

    EXTREMITIES: Extremities reveal no edema.

IMPRESSION: Intraductal carcinoma, upper outer quadrant, right breast

PLAN: The patient came back to the office yesterday morning with her husband. The situation was explained to them. Since this is an intraductal carcinoma in situ, Lumpectomy will be performed and sentinel node dissection will be carried out. Whether the patient needs further treatment or not depends on the findings of the permanent sections of the specimen. The patient and her husband understand the situation very well and agreed to proceed with surgery.

OPERATIVE REPORT—PATIENT 1

PREOPERATIVE DIAGNOSIS: Intraductal carcinoma in situ, upper outer quadrant, right breast

POSTOPERATIVE DIAGNOSIS: Intraductal carcinoma in situ, upper outer quadrant, right breast

OPERATION: Lumpectomy and sentinel right axillary lymph node dissection

ANESTHESIA: General anesthesia with laryngeal intubation

PROCEDURE: After obtaining the informed consent, the patient was brought into the operating room and placed on the table in the supine position. General anesthesia with laryngeal intubation was conducted smoothly. The skin over the right chest and right arm was prepped and draped in the usual sterile manner. The intended incision line was marked with a marking pen. The radioactive isotope for the sentinel node dissection was injected. The breast tissue was massaged. Five minutes were then allowed to pass before the incision was made.

The incision was made with excision of the previous incisional scar. The lymphatics were identified and dissected. The suspicious right axillary sentinel nodes were dissected. Then the lumpectomy was performed with upper and lower skin flaps. The dissection of the breast tissue and subcutaneous tissue to raise the two flaps was conducted smoothly. A large lump was dissected and the dissection carried to the pectoralis muscles. The big lump was removed completely. Hemostasis was confirmed by cauterization. The wound was then irrigated with copious amounts of warm water solution. The specimen was sent to pathology and the sentinel nodes were sent separately to pathology. The wound was then closed in layers using 2-0 Vicryl for the deeper layer, 3-0 Vicryl for the subcutaneous tissue, and 4-0 Vicryl for the skin.

The patient tolerated the whole procedure very well and was sent to the recovery room in stable condition after extubation.

Blood loss was minimal. Sponge and needle counts were correct. No drain was left. The specimens were sent to pathology.

Exam 1 Case Studies

PATHOLOGY REPORT—PATIENT 1

DATE: 8/3

SPECIMEN: Breast lump and lymph node

GROSS DESCRIPTION: The specimen is submitted as breast and lymphatic tissue. It consists of breast tissue measuring 2.0 cm, 1.5 cm, 1.0 cm.

DIAGNOSIS: Intraductal carcinoma in situ

Choose the correct principal diagnosis code.

- a. C50.221
- b. C50.411
- c. D05.11
- d. D05.82
- e. D05.92

Choose the correct secondary diagnosis code(s).

- a. E03.9
- b. E11.9
- c. E11.22
- d. E78.2
- e. E78.5
- f. I10
- g. I12.9
- h. R03.0
- i. R73.9
- j. None apply

Choose the correct procedure code(s).

- a. 19300-LT
- b. 19301-RT
- c. 19302
- d. 19303
- e. 19305-RT
- f. 19307-LT
- g. 38525
- h. 38530
- i. 38790
- j. 38792

SAME-DAY SURGERY SUMMARY—PATIENT 2

HISTORY AND PHYSICAL EXAMINATION

DATE: 1/29

HISTORY OF PRESENT ILLNESS: This is a 62-year-old male with progressive painful blurring of vision due to aphakic bullous keratopathy with moderate stage glaucoma in the left eye. He has undergone previous Molteno implant with poor vision and pain due to ruptured bulla. The patient is admitted for transplant at this time.

PAST MEDICAL HISTORY: The patient has angina and COPD. There have been no recent episodes of chest pain or shortness of breath. The patient also underwent a prostatectomy six years ago for prostatic carcinoma.

ALLERGIES: None known

CHRONIC MEDICATIONS: Ventolin and nitroglycerin as needed for chest pain

SOCIAL HISTORY: The patient is a 62-year-old male who is married and lives with his wife. He has 5 grandchildren. He is a nondrinker and a nonsmoker.

REVIEW OF SYSTEMS: The patient has normal bowels. He has had no problems with his urine since his prostatectomy. There is no hematuria or dysuria. The patient has had two colds in the past six weeks. He states that he has been having some difficulty sleeping because of the pain in his shoulder. This has limited some of the activity that he normally does, such as golf.

PHYSICAL EXAMINATION: This is a well-developed, well-nourished 62-year-old male who appears younger than his stated age.

HEENT: Aphakic post-cataract extraction, neck supple

CHEST: The lungs are clear to percussion and auscultation. The heart has normal rhythm and pulse.

ABDOMEN: Abdomen reveals no masses; bowel sounds are heard.

EXTREMITIES: Extremities reveal no edema.

OPERATIVE REPORT—PATIENT 2

PREOPERATIVE DIAGNOSES:

1. Aphakic bullous keratopathy left eye
2. Open-angle glaucoma left eye
3. Chronic iritis bilateral

POSTOPERATIVE DIAGNOSES:

1. Aphakic bullous keratopathy left eye
2. Open-angle glaucoma left eye
3. Chronic iritis bilateral

OPERATION:

1. Aphakic penetrating keratoplasty left eye
2. Posterior chamber intraocular lens scleral implant left eye
3. Open-sky mechanical automated vitrectomy left eye

ANESTHESIA: Retrobulbar block, monitored anesthesia care

COMPLICATIONS: None

INDICATIONS: This is a 62-year-old gentleman with progressive painful blurring of vision due to aphakic bullous keratopathy following cataract extraction, also with glaucoma. He has undergone previous Molteno implant with poor vision and pain due to ruptured bulla. The patient is admitted for transplant at this time. After informed consent, the patient agreed to the benefits and risks of surgery.

PROCEDURE DESCRIPTION: The patient was taken to the operating room. Under monitored anesthesia care, he was given a retrobulbar block in the standard fashion for a total of 4 cc of a 50/50 mixture 0.75% Marcaine and 4% lidocaine with Wydase.

After ensuring adequate anesthesia as well as akinesia, the patient was prepped and draped in the usual sterile ophthalmologic fashion. A wire lid speculum was inserted, and a small conjunctival peritomy was made at the two o'clock and ten o'clock hour positions to prepare for half-thickness scleral flaps for suturing a scleral-supported lens in the left eye. A Flieringa ring was then attached in the standard fashion using four interrupted 5-0 Dacron sutures. Attention was then placed to the back Mayo, and a 7.75-mm donor button was harvested, epithelial side down, in the standard fashion. Routine surveillance cultures were sent, and the donor button was placed on the Mayo stand in a Petri dish. Attention was then placed on the donor's cornea, and using a Barron-Hessburg trephine device, a 7.50-mm button was harvested under viscoelastic support. Corneoscleral scissors were used to the left and right respectively to remove the button in toto. Vitrectomy was then performed due to prolapsing vitreous, and an attempt to reposition the iris was made. However, due to loss of iris material during prior surgeries, I was unable to close the sphincter defect. After completing the vitrectomy, a scleral-supported CZ70VD 7-mm lens was secured using a 10-0 Prolene suture at the ten and two o'clock hour positions. Scleral flaps were then closed over the 10-0 Prolene to maintain a tight closure. The button was then sewn into position using 16 interrupted 10-0 nylon sutures in the standard fashion. All the knots were cut short and buried in the recipient side of the host junction. A final check to make sure the chamber was watertight was unremarkable, and the Flieringa ring was removed followed by the bridle sutures. Subconjunctival Ancef and Celestone were placed, and a bandage contact lens was placed on the eye.

The patient was taken to the recovery room in good repair without complications of the above procedure.

Choose the correct principal diagnosis code.

   a. H16.231
   b. H18.12
   c. H18.221
   d. H59.012
   e. H59.019

Choose the correct secondary diagnosis code(s).

   a. H20.10
   b. H20.13
   c. H27.02
   d. H40.10X2
   e. I20.9
   f. I25.110
   g. I25.119
   h. J44.0
   i. J44.9
   j. None apply

Choose the correct procedure code(s).

   a. 65710-RT
   b. 65730
   c. 65750-LT
   d. 65755-LT
   e. 65757
   f. 66982-RT
   g. 66985-LT
   h. 66986
   i. 67005-50
   j. 67010-LT

EMERGENCY DEPARTMENT RECORD—PATIENT 3

DATE OF ADMISSION: 6/17   **DATE OF DISCHARGE:** 6/17

HISTORY (Problem Focused):

ADMISSION HISTORY: This is a 29-year-old Asian female. She was walking down her steps when she fell. The patient complains of pain in the right arm.

ALLERGIES: Penicillin

CHRONIC MEDICATIONS: Normally takes no drugs but has been taking ibuprofen every 6 hours because of painful arm.

FAMILY HISTORY: Noncontributory

SOCIAL HISTORY: The patient smokes one pack of cigarettes per day. She drinks one drink per day.

REVIEW OF SYSTEMS: The patient had hives the last time she took penicillin. Her cardiovascular, genitourinary, and gastrointestinal systems are negative.

PHYSICAL EXAMINATION (Expanded Problem Focused):

GENERAL APPEARANCE: This is an alert cooperative female in no acute distress.

HEENT: PERRLA, extraocular movements are full

NECK: Supple

CHEST: Lungs are clear. Heart has normal sinus rhythm.

ABDOMEN: Soft and nontender, no organomegaly

EXTREMITIES: Examination of the arm reveals painful movement.

LABORATORY AND X-RAY DATA: Urinalysis is normal; EKG normal; chest x-ray is normal; CBC and diff show no abnormalities; x-ray of the right arm revealed a fracture of the shaft of the humerus.

IMPRESSION: Fracture of the mid-shaft of the right humerus

PLAN: Reduction fracture of the humerus

TREATMENT: Following administration of conscious sedation, the patient's humeral fracture was reduced and a cast applied. One fracture tray was used.

DISCHARGE DIAGNOSIS: Fracture of the shaft of the right humerus

INSTRUCTIONS ON DISCHARGE: The patient is instructed to make an appointment with the orthopedic clinic in 3 days, to take one Percocet every 4 hours as needed for pain as per the label. Call the ER doctor if swelling or blue color of the fingers occurs. The patient is also counseled to stop smoking and was instructed to make an appointment with her primary care physician to discuss smoking cessation.

Code the procedures that are done in the emergency department as well as the facility E/M code based on the point values, CPT codes and table below.

Emergency Department E/M Level Point Value Key

Level 1 = 1–20

Level 2 = 21–35

Level 3 = 36–47

Level 4 = 48–60

Level 5 = > 61

Critical Care > 61 with constant physician attendance

CPT Codes Corresponding to Emergency Department E/M Level

Level 1	99281	99281–25 with procedure/laboratory/radiology
Level 2	99282	99282–25 with procedure/laboratory/radiology
Level 3	99283	99283–25 with procedure/laboratory/radiology
Level 4	99284	99284–25 with procedure/laboratory/radiology
Level 5	99285	99285–25 with procedure/laboratory/radiology

Emergency Department Acuity Points					
	5	10	15	20	25
Number of Meds Given	1–2	3–5	6–7	8–9	> 10
Extent of Hx	Brief	PF	EPF	Detail	Comprehensive
Extent of Examination	Brief	PF	EPF	Detail	Comprehensive
Number of Tests Ordered	0–1	2–3	4–5	6–7	> 8
Number of Supplies Used	1	2–3	4–5	6–7	> 8

Choose the correct principal diagnosis code.

a. S42.251A

b. S42.254A

c. S42.301A

d. S42.311A

e. S42.321A

Choose the correct secondary diagnosis code(s).

a. E03.9
b. E11.9
c. E78.5
d. F17.210
e. I10
f. I50.9
g. I25.10
h. I25.119
i. K21.9
j. J44.9
k. None apply

Choose the correct procedure code(s).

a. 24500
b. 24505-RT
c. 24515-LT
d. 24516-RT
e. 24530
f. 24535-RT
g. 24538-LT
h. 99282-27
i. 99283-23
j. 99284-25

AMBULATORY RECORD—PATIENT 4

Right and left heart catheterization and coronary angiography

PROCEDURE: After obtaining informed consent the patient was taken to the cardiac catheterization laboratory. The right groin was prepped and draped in the usual fashion and 2% Xylocaine was used to anesthetize. 6-French sheaths were introduced into the right femoral artery and vein and a 6-French multipurpose catheter was used for the heart catheterization, coronary angiography, and ventricular angiography. Right heart pressures and cardiac outputs were measured. A pigtail catheter was inserted into the left ventricular cavity and ventricular pressures obtained. Angiography of the right coronary artery was performed. Left ventricular angiography and aortic root angiography was performed. The patient tolerated the procedure well without complications.

DIAGNOSIS: Arteriosclerotic coronary artery disease

Choose the correct principal diagnosis code.

- a. I25.10
- b. I25.110
- c. I25.111
- d. I25.118
- e. I25.119

Choose the correct secondary diagnosis code(s).

- a. E10.9
- b. E78.2
- c. E78.5
- d. F17.290
- e. I10
- f. I50.9
- g. K21.9
- h. K57.30
- i. J44.9
- j. None apply

Choose the correct procedure code(s).

- a. 93451
- b. 93452
- c. 93453
- d. 93454
- e. 93456
- f. 93460
- g. 93563
- h. 93564
- i. 93565
- j. 93567

Exam 1 Case Studies

INPATIENT RECORD—PATIENT 5

DISCHARGE SUMMARY

DATE OF ADMISSION: 2/3   **DATE OF DISCHARGE:** 2/5

DISCHARGE DIAGNOSIS: Full-term pregnancy—delivered liveborn male infant

Patient started labor spontaneously three days before her due date. She was brought to the hospital by automobile. Labor progressed for a while but then contractions became fewer and she delivered soon after. A midline episiotomy was done. Membranes and placenta were complete. There was some bleeding but not excessively. Patient made an uneventful recovery.

HISTORY AND PHYSICAL EXAMINATION—PATIENT 5

ADMITTED: 2/3

REASON FOR ADMISSION: Full-term pregnancy at 38 weeks

PAST MEDICAL HISTORY: Previous deliveries normal and mitral valve prolapse

ALLERGIES: None known

CHRONIC MEDICATIONS: None

FAMILY HISTORY: Heart disease—father

SOCIAL HISTORY: The patient is married and has one other child living with her.

REVIEW OF SYSTEMS:

    SKIN: Normal

    HEAD-SCALP: Normal

    EYES: Normal

    ENT: Normal

    NECK: Normal

    BREASTS: Normal

    THORAX: Normal

    LUNGS: Normal

    HEART: Slight midsystolic click with late systolic murmur II/VI

    ABDOMEN: Normal

IMPRESSION: Good health with term pregnancy. History of mitral valve prolapse—asymptomatic.

PROGRESS NOTES—PATIENT 5

DATE	NOTE
2/3	Admit to Labor and Delivery. MVP stable. Patient progressing well. Delivered at 1:15 p.m. one full-term male infant.
2/4	Patient doing well. Mitral valve prolapse stable. The perineum is clean and dry, incision intact.
2/5	Will discharge to home

PHYSICIAN'S ORDERS—PATIENT 5

DATE	ORDER
2/3	Admit to Labor and Delivery 1,000 cc 5% D/LR May ambulate Type and screen CBC May have ice chips
2/5	Discharge patient to home.

DELIVERY RECORD—PATIENT 5

DATE: 2/3

The patient was 3 cm dilated when admitted. The duration of the first stage of labor was 6 hours, second stage was 14 minutes, third stage was 5 minutes. She was given local anesthesia. An episiotomy was performed with repair. There were no lacerations. The cord was wrapped once around the baby's neck, but did not cause compression. The mother and liveborn baby were discharged from the delivery room in good condition.

Exam 1 Case Studies

LABORATORY REPORT—PATIENT 5

HEMATOLOGY

DATE: 2/3

Specimen	Results	Normal Values
WBC	5.2	4.3–11.0
RBC	4.9	4.5–5.9
HGB	13.8	13.5–17.5
HCT	45	41–52
MCV	93	80–100
MCHC	41	31–57
PLT	255	150–450

Choose the correct principal diagnosis code.

   a. O69.0XX0
   b. O69.1XX0
   c. O69.81X0
   d. O69.89X0
   e. O80

Choose the correct secondary diagnosis code(s).

   a. O99.283
   b. O99.284
   c. O99.413
   d. O99.42
   e. I34.0
   f. I34.1
   g. Z37.0
   h. Z37.1
   i. Z3A.38
   j. None apply

Choose the correct procedure code(s).

a. 10D00Z0
b. 10D07Z3
c. 10D07Z7
d. 10E0XZZ
e. 0W0M0ZZ
f. 0W0M37Z
g. 0W0N0JZ
h. 0W0N0KZ
i. 0W8NXZZ
j. 0WMN0ZZ

INPATIENT RECORD—PATIENT 6

DISCHARGE SUMMARY

DATE OF ADMISSION: 1/31   **DATE OF DISCHARGE:** 2/3

DISCHARGE DIAGNOSIS: Right lower lobe pneumonia due to gram-negative bacteria, resistant to erythromycin

ADMISSION HISTORY: This is a 56-year-old insulin-requiring diabetic female whose diabetes is out of control whom we have been following for hypertension, degenerative joint disease, aortic stenosis and diabetic retinopathy. Over the past three days she has noted increased cough and chest congestion with a fever of approximately 102 degrees. She was found to have a right lower lobe infiltrate and was started on therapy with erythromycin. Despite initial therapy, the patient's clinical status has worsened over the past 24 hours.

COURSE IN HOSPITAL: Patient was admitted with the diagnosis of right lower lobe pneumonia. She was begun on intravenous ceftriaxone. Because of difficulties with venous access, patient was switched to intramuscular ceftriaxone on her third hospital day.

By 2/3 the patient was afebrile and her cough had diminished. Her blood pressure was well controlled at 140/74.

INSTRUCTIONS ON DISCHARGE: Follow up with me by phone in three days and in my office in two weeks. Repeat chest x-ray to be done then.

MEDICATIONS:

1. Calan SR 180 mg b.i.d.
2. Zestril 20 mg PO q. a.m.
3. NPH Insulin, 30 units, sub q., a.m.
4. Levoquin 500 mg PO daily ×10 days
5. Celebrex 100 mg PO b.i.d.

HISTORY AND PHYSICAL EXAMINATION—PATIENT 6

ADMITTED: 1/31

REASON FOR ADMISSION: Physical examination on admission revealed a well-developed, acutely ill-appearing black female.

HISTORY OF PRESENT ILLNESS: A 56-year-old diabetic followed for hypertension and diabetic retinopathy. Over the past three days she has noted increased cough and chest congestion with a fever of approximately 102 degrees. She was found to have a right lower lobe infiltrate and was begun on therapy with erythromycin. Despite initial therapy, the patient's clinical status worsened over the past 24 hours and hospitalization was recommended.

PAST MEDICAL HISTORY: Hypertension, degenerative joint disease in both knees, and moderate aortic stenosis

ALLERGIES: Dust

CHRONIC MEDICATIONS: Calan SR 180 mg po b.i.d., Insulin (NPH), Zestril 20 mg PO daily, Celebrex 100 mg PO b.i.d.

FAMILY HISTORY: Notable for hypertension in mother

SOCIAL HISTORY: Noncontributory

PHYSICAL EXAMINATION:

    GENERAL APPEARANCE: The patient is a well-developed black female in moderate distress.

    VITAL SIGNS: T 102, P 80, R 16, BP 150/80

    SKIN: Warm and dry

    HEENT: Significant for mildly inflamed mucous membranes. Retinopathy evident in both eyes.

    NECK: Supple. Symmetrical with no bruits

    LUNGS: Coarse rhonchi bilaterally, right greater than left

    HEART: Regular rate and rhythm, positive S1, positive III/VI SEM

    ABDOMEN: Soft, nontender, no mass

GENITALIA: Deferred

RECTAL: Deferred

EXTREMITIES: No edema

NEUROLOGIC: Normal

Exam 1 Case Studies

HISTORY AND PHYSICAL EXAMINATION—PATIENT 6

LABORATORY DATA:

1. EKG: NSR, widespread ST-T wave abnormalities, LV hypertrophy
2. CBC: Hgb 13, Hct 38, WBC 12.8
3. Glucose: 281
4. Urinalysis: Unremarkable
5. Sputum: Gram stain—a few WBCs, moderate gram-negative rods

IMPRESSION:

1. Right lower lobe pneumonia possibly due to gram-negative bacteria
2. Diabetes mellitus on insulin—uncontrolled
3. Hypertension—stable
4. Degenerative joint disease—stable
5. Moderate aortic stenosis

PLAN: Admit, IV antibiotics for pneumonia. Monitor blood sugars.

PROGRESS NOTES—PATIENT 6

DATE	NOTE
1/31	Patient admitted for cough associated with increased temperature with chest x-ray indicative of pneumonia. Will obtain sputum culture and begin on ceftriaxone. Will monitor blood pressure and blood sugars. Will use sliding scale to bring blood sugar into control. Patient with recent echocardiogram as outpatient that showed stable aortic stenosis.
2/1	The patient is responding well. Will request diabetic education nurse to meet with her and set up an appointment for classes following this admission.
2/2	Sputum culture reveals gram-negative bacteria as suspected. Patient's temperature is down. Patient resting comfortably. Blood sugar better.
2/3	Blood sugar with increasing control today. The importance of appropriate diet emphasized. Will discharge with p.o. antibiotics.

PHYSICIAN'S ORDERS—PATIENT 6

DATE	ORDER
1/31/20XX	Admit to 3 South
	DX: Pneumonia
	Please give ceftriaxone 1 g q 8 hours IV
	ADA diet
	CBC and SMA
	Calan SR 50 mg in a.m. with orange juice
	Zestril 2 in a.m.
	Celebrex 100 mg po BID
	Accu-Chek before meals and before bedtime
	Chest x-ray
	Sliding scale for insulin as follows:
	Below 120 give 4 units of regular
	120–200 give 6 units of regular insulin
	200–300 give 8 units of regular insulin
	Above 300, call physician
2/1/20XX	Change insulin to 40 NPH units sq in a.m. today.
	Consult diabetic nurse to see patient and set up classes following admission.
2/2/20XX	Continue insulin to 40 NPH units sq in a.m. today.
2/2/20XX	D/C IV and switch to ceftriaxone 1 g IM q. 24 hrs
2/3/20XX	Discharge to home.

Exam 1 Case Studies

LABORATORY REPORTS—PATIENT 6

MICROBIOLOGY

DATE	TEST TYPE	
1/31/20XX	SOURCE:	
	SITE:	
	GRAM STAIN RESULTS: Sputum	
	CULTURE RESULTS: Slight WBCs, Slight Epis	
	Many gram-negative rods	
	sl. gram-negative diplococci	
	sl. gram-positive cocci in clusters	
	SUSCEPTIBILITY:	S
	AMPICILLIN	S
	CEFAZOLIN	S
	CEFOTAXIME	S
	CEFTRIAXONE	S
	CEFUROXIME	S
	CEPHALOTHIN	S
	CIPROFLOXACIN	S
	ERYTHROMYCIN	R
	GENTAMICIN	S
	OXACILLIN	S
	PENICILLIN	S
	PIPERACILLIN	S
	TETRACYCLINE	S
	TOBRAMYCIN	S
	TRIMETH/SULF	S
	VANCOMYCIN	S

S = SUSCEPTIBLE

R = RESISTANT

I = INTERMEDIATE

M = MODERATELY SUSCEP

RADIOLOGY REPORT—PATIENT 6

DATE: 1/31/20XX

HISTORY DIAGNOSIS: Pneumonia

FINDINGS: There is slight overexpansion of the lungs. The pulmonary vasculature is normal. The heart is not enlarged. There is lower lobe infiltrate in the right lung.

IMPRESSION: Right lower lobe pneumonia

EKG REPORT—PATIENT 6

DATE: 1/31/20XX

DIAGNOSIS: Pneumonia

INTERPRETATION: EKG: NSR, widespread ST-T wave abnormalities, LV hypertrophy

LABORATORY REPORT—PATIENT 6

CHEMISTRY

DATE: 1/31/20XX

Specimen	Results	Normal Values
GLUC	281 H	70–110
CREAT	0.67	0.5–1.5
NA	142	136–146
K	4.8	3.5–5.5
CL	108	95–110
CO_2	29	24–32
CA	9.5	8.4–10.5
PHOS	3.8	2.5–4.4
MG	2.8	1.6–3.0
T BILI	1.0	0.2–1.2
D BILI	0.3	0.0–0.5
PROTEIN	6.5	6.0–8.0
ALBUMIN	5.1	5.0–5.5
AST	38	0–40
ALT	54	30–65
GGT	50	15–85
LD	180	100–190
ALK PHOS	102	50–136
URIC ACID	4.5	2.2–7.7
CHOL	89	0–200
TRIG	101	10–160

LABORATORY REPORT—PATIENT 6 (continued)

URINALYSIS—PATIENT 6

DATE: 1/31

Test	Result	Ref Range
SP GRAVITY	1.007	1.005–1.035
PH	7.0	5–7
PROT	NEG	NEG
GLUC	NEG	NEG
KETONES	NEG	NEG
BILI	NEG	NEG
BLOOD	NEG	NEG
LEU EST	NEG	NEG
NITRATES	NEG	NEG
RED SUBS	NEG	NEG

HEMATOLOGY—PATIENT 6

DATE: 1/31

Specimen	Results	Normal Values
WBC	12.8 H	4.3–11.0
RBC	5.5	4.5–5.9
HGB	13.0 L	13.5–17.5
HCT	38 L	41–52
MCV	90	80–100
MCHC	41	31–57
PLT	251	150–450

BLOOD GLUCOSE MONITORING RECORD—PATIENT 6

1/31/20XX	11:00 a.m.	310
	4:00 p.m.	300
	9:00 p.m.	290
2/1/20XX	7:00 a.m.	150
	11:00 a.m.	175
	4:00 p.m.	145
	9:00 p.m.	175
2/2/20XX	7:00 a.m.	140
	11:00 a.m.	135
	4:00 p.m.	160
	9:00 p.m.	150
2/3/20XX	7:00 a.m.	135
	11:00 a.m.	150
	4:00 p.m.	130

Choose the correct principal diagnosis code.

a. E11.65
b. I10
c. I12.9
d. J15.6
e. K21.9

Choose the correct secondary diagnosis code(s).

a. E11.311
b. E11.319
c. E10.65
d. E11.65
e. I10
f. I35.0
g. M17.0
h. Z16.29
i. Z79.4
j. None apply

Choose the correct procedure code(s).

a. 0T9B00Z
b. 0T9B80Z
c. 30233K1
d. 30233R1
e. 30243N0
f. 4A023N7
g. 4A1Z7KZ
h. 4A197LZ
i. 4A1971Z
j. None apply

INPATIENT RECORD—PATIENT 7

DISCHARGE SUMMARY

DATE OF ADMISSION: 1/3   **DATE OF DISCHARGE:** 1/7

DISCHARGE DIAGNOSIS: Recurrent carcinoma, left lung

This is a 63-year-old female who is two years status post left upper lobe resection for adenocarcinoma. Pathology at that time revealed a positive bronchial margin of resection. She was treated with postop radiation and has done extremely well. She has remained asymptomatic with no postoperative difficulty. Follow-up serial CT scans have revealed a new lesion in the apical portion of the left lung, which on needle biopsy was positive for adenocarcinoma. She was admitted specifically for a left thoracotomy and possible pneumonectomy.

PAST MEDICAL HISTORY: Positive for tobacco abuse 2 PPD × 30 years in the past. Significant for a right parotidectomy and also significant for hypertension, degenerative joint disease of lumbar spine, and chronic pulmonary disease. The patient also suffered a stroke in the left brain with resulting right hemiparesis three years ago. Medications on discharge: Tenormin 25 mg once a day, Calan SR 240 mg twice a day, Moduretic one tablet q. day and K-Dur 10 meq q. day, Proventil MDI 2 puffs PO q.i.d. p.r.n., Azacort MDI 2 puffs PO t.i.d., Vioxx 25 mg PO daily.

PHYSICAL EXAMINATION: Revealed a well-healed right parotid incision. No supraclavicular adenopathy. She has a healed left posterior lateral thoracotomy scar. Impression is that of local recurrence, status post left upper lobectomy. She is to undergo a left pneumonectomy.

OPERATIVE FINDINGS AND HOSPITAL COURSE: There was a large mass in the remaining lung, extensive mediastinal fibrosis, bronchial margin free by frozen section. Following surgery she was placed in the intensive care unit postoperatively. The chest tube was removed on postoperative day number two.

She experienced some EKG changes consistent with acute nontransmural MI. Cardiology was consulted, and she was started on nitroglycerin and IV heparin. She was eventually weaned from her oxygen therapy.

She was started on regular diet and was discharged in good condition. Her wound was clean and dry.

INSTRUCTIONS ON DISCHARGE: Discharged home with instructions to follow up with cardiology next week. Also follow up with me in the office.

HISTORY AND PHYSICAL EXAMINATION—PATIENT 7

ADMITTED: 1/3

HISTORY OF PRESENT ILLNESS: Patient is a 63-year-old right-handed female with history of adenocarcinoma of apical segment of left upper lobe of lung, now presenting with mass of left lower lobe. She has received radiation therapy to her chest. She weighs 123 pounds. She also has chronic obstructive pulmonary disease.

REVIEW OF SYSTEMS: She can climb two flights of steps with minimal difficulties. She has a significant underbite. She has stiffness in lower spine, worse in the a.m. She has hypertension and took her Tenormin 25 mg, Calan SR 240 mg this a.m.

PAST SURGICAL HISTORY: She had a right parotidectomy seven years ago and was told they needed to use a "very small" ETT. Two years ago she underwent a left upper lobe resection at this facility. Previous medical records are being requested.

ALLERGIES: She is allergic to sulfa. Postoperatively last time she received Demerol. She also had hallucinations in the ICU for several days. She blames the hallucinations on the Demerol. The only allergy sign was hallucinations.

PHYSICAL EXAMINATION: Revealed a well-healed right parotid incision. No supraclavicular adenopathy. She has a healed left posterior lateral thoracotomy scar. Impression is that of local recurrence, status post left upper lobectomy. She is to undergo a left completion pneumonectomy, muscle flap coverage of bronchial stump. The patient has hemiparesis in the right extremities.

IMPRESSION: Carcinoma left lower lobe of lung

PLAN: Pneumonectomy of left lung. The patient is agreeable to general endotracheal anesthesia or the use of epidural narcotic. She is agreeable to postoperative ventilation if necessary.

PROGRESS NOTES—PATIENT 7

DATE	NOTE
1/3	Attending Physician: Admit for recurrent lung carcinoma, s/p radiation therapy. Consent signed for pneumonectomy. Epidural morphine usage postop explained to and discussed with the patient. She is agreeable.
	Anesthesia Preop: Patient evaluated and examined. General anesthesia chosen. Patient agrees. Will provide postop epidural morphine for pain management s/p thoracotomy.
	Attending Physician:
	Procedure Note:
	Preop Dx: Local recurrence of carcinoma of the lung
	Postop Dx: Same
	Procedure: Pneumonectomy with muscle flap coverage of bronchial stump
	Complications: R/O Intraop MI
	Anesthesia Postop: Patient in stable condition following GEA with possible intraoperative MI due to hypotension. CPK to be evaluated as available. Patient comfortable with epidural morphine. No adverse effects of anesthesia experienced.
1/4	Attending Physician: Path report confirms recurrent adenocarcinoma. Patient stable but with persistent hypotension resolving slowly—will consult cardiology. CPK MB positive. Incision clean and dry. COPD stable, arthritis stable.
	Cardiology Consult: The patient has resolving intraoperative myocardial infarction due to demand ischemia caused by the hypotension. Will continue to monitor.
1/5	Attending Physician: Looks and feels well, weaning off morphine. Blood pressure stable. Left pleural space expanding and filling space. Chest tube removed, epidural cath removed.
	Cardiology Consult: The patient looking and feeling better.
1/6	Attending Physician: Patient stable for discharge in a.m. Cardiology to follow.

OPERATIVE REPORT—PATIENT 7

DATE: 1/3

OPERATION: Pneumonectomy

PREOPERATIVE DIAGNOSIS: Recurrent carcinoma of left lung

POSTOPERATIVE DIAGNOSIS: Same

ANESTHESIA: General endotracheal anesthesia

OPERATIVE FINDINGS: There was a large mass in the left lower lobe.

The patient was prepped and draped in the usual fashion. Following thoracotomy the left lung was completely removed. A muscle flap coverage was used for the bronchial stump. During the procedure the patient experienced an episode of hypotension, watch for resulting MI. The patient was fluid resuscitated and sent to the recovery room in good condition.

PATHOLOGY REPORT—PATIENT 7

DATE: 1/3

SPECIMEN: Left lung, resected

CLINICAL DATA: This is a 63-year-old female with recurrent disease on CT scan.

DIAGNOSIS: Adenocarcinoma of the lower lobe of the left lung, bronchial margin is free of disease.

PHYSICIAN'S ORDERS—PATIENT 7

DATE	ORDER
1/3	Admit to surgical floor
	Standard orders for thoracotomy
	Tenormin 25 mg q.d.
	Calan SR 240 mg twice a day
	Moduretic one tab. q.d.
	K-Dur 10 meq q.d. in a.m.
	Vioxx 25 mg PO daily in a.m.
	Proventil (albuterol) MDI 2 puffs PO q.i.d.
	Azmacort MDI 2 puffs PO q.i.d.
	CBC
	Postop Orders:
	Admit to ICU
	Serial CPK stat
	CBC
	SMA 12
	Anesthesia:
	Morphine pump ad lib
	D5NSS 100 cc/hr
	Strict input and output documentation
1/4	Attending MD: Consult Cardiology
	Cardiology: Lasix 20 mg b.i.d. PO
	D/C IV
1/5	Transfer to floor
	Continue meds
1/6	Discharge patient in a.m.

LABORATORY REPORTS—PATIENT 7

HEMATOLOGY

DATE: 1/3

Specimen	Results	Normal Values
WBC	5.7	4.3–11.0
RBC	5.0	4.5–5.9
HGB	15.6	13.5–17.5
HCT	47	41–52
MCV	89	80–100
MCHC	42	31–57
PLT	300	150–450

HEMATOLOGY—PATIENT 7

DATE: 1/4

Specimen	Results	Normal Values
WBC	5.6	4.3–11.0
RBC	4.0 L	4.5–5.9
HGB	13.4 L	13.5–17.5
HCT	40 L	41–52
MCV	82	80–100
MCHC	33	31–57
PLT	200	150–450

LABORATORY REPORTS—PATIENT 7 (continued)

CHEMISTRY—PATIENT 7

DATE: 1/3

Specimen	Results	Normal Values
GLUC	90	70–110
BUN	27 H	8–25
CREAT	1.0	0.5–1.5
NA	138	136–146
K	4.0	3.5–5.5
CL	100	95–110
CO_2	28	24–32
CA	8.9	8.4–10.5
PHOS	2.9	2.5–4.4
MG	2.0	1.6–3.0
T BILI	1.0	0.2–1.2
D BILI	0.04	0.0–0.5
PROTEIN	7.0	6.0–8.0
ALBUMIN	5.3	5.0–5.5
AST	35	0–40
ALT	50	30–65
MB	7 H, 15 H, 12 H, 9 H	0–5.0
CPK	221, 250 H, 275 H, 230	21–232

RADIOLOGY REPORT—PATIENT 7

DATE: 1/3

CHEST X-RAY: Reveals mass in the left lower lobe. There are surgical clips in the thorax from apparent previous surgery. The thoracic organs are midline and the vasculature is normal.

IMPRESSION: Carcinoma LLL, no congestive heart failure.

RADIOLOGY REPORT—PATIENT 7

DATE: 1/4

CHEST X-RAY: Reveals absence of left lung. Other architecture is normal other than postoperative changes. The thoracic organs are midline and the vasculature is normal.

IMPRESSION: Postop changes consistent with lobectomy; no congestive heart failure.

EKG REPORT—PATIENT 7

DATE: 1/3

Normal sinus rhythm

DATE: 1/4

There are nonspecific ST changes consistent with possible evolving myocardial infarction due to demand ischemia as a result of the intraoperative hypotension.

DATE: 1/5

Possible acute myocardial infarction, please correlate with other clinical findings.

Choose the correct principal diagnosis code.

   a. C34.32
   b. C34.82
   c. I95.89
   d. I97.791
   e. J44.9

Choose the correct secondary diagnosis code(s).

   a. C34.32
   b. I10
   c. I21.A1
   d. I69.351
   e. I95.89
   f. I97.791
   g. J44.9
   h. M47.816
   i. Z87.891
   j. Z92.3

Choose the correct procedure code(s) that apply.

   a. 0BBF0ZZ
   b. 0BBJ0ZZ
   c. 0BCF3ZZ
   d. 0BCB8ZZ
   e. 0BCJ0ZZ
   f. 0BDB8ZX
   g. 0BDL4ZX
   h. 0BTB0ZZ
   i. 0BTL0ZZ
   j. None apply

INPATIENT RECORD—PATIENT 8

DISCHARGE SUMMARY

DATE OF ADMISSION: 4/19   **DATE OF DISCHARGE:** 4/24

DISCHARGE DIAGNOSIS:

    Acute inferior wall myocardial infarction (STEMI)

    Hyperlipidemia

    Complete heart block

    Upper gastrointestinal hemorrhage

    Arteriosclerotic heart disease

ADMISSION HISTORY: This is a 45-year-old white male with a history of hyperlipidemia and tobacco use. He presented to the hospital with an acute myocardial infarction. He was treated with peripheral intravenous TPA and had a reperfusion. The patient continued to have chest pain with an inferior ST elevation on EKG.

COURSE IN HOSPITAL: The patient sustained an acute myocardial infarction. The patient presented with an acute myocardial infarction and underwent catheterization. The patient was found to have stenosis of the mid-right coronary artery and right distal coronary artery. The left coronary branches have minimal noncritical disease. The left ventricular ejection fraction was approximately 45% with inferior wall hypokinesis.

The patient had a successful PTCA to the mid-RCA with a stent. I initially attempted to dilate with a balloon, but the results were inadequate and proceeded to place a 4.0-mm J&J stent. The patient continued to have anginal symptomatology and for this reason was taken to the OR for CABG ×2. He did well after the CABG ×2 without any anginal symptoms.

The patient also had gastrointestinal bleeding following the PTCA. The patient developed retching and hematemesis and anemia for which he required blood transfusion. The probable cause of the nausea and vomiting was a reaction to anesthesia. Upper endoscopy revealed no evidence of peptic ulcer disease.

At the present time the patient has been treated with aspirin and Ticlid and has been doing very well. The plan is to discharge him home with follow-up in my office next week.

INSTRUCTIONS ON DISCHARGE: Follow up in 1 week in my office. Medications include; aspirin 1 tablet per day, Ticlid 250 mg twice per day, Tagamet 400 mg twice per day and sublingual nitroglycerin as needed for chest pain. Condition upon discharge is stable. Activity is restricted until cardiac rehabilitation.

HISTORY AND PHYSICAL EXAMINATION—PATIENT 8

ADMITTED: 4/19

    Acute inferior wall myocardial infarction (STEMI)

    Complete heart block

    Ventricular ectopy

    Possible ASHD

REASON FOR ADMISSION: Pain in chest

HISTORY OF PRESENT ILLNESS: This is a pleasant 45-year-old male with a history of hyperlipidemia and previous tobacco use. He also has a family history of coronary artery disease. He denies any prior history of coronary artery disease, myocardial infarction, or CVAs. The patient has been essentially very healthy, except for occasional skipped heartbeat in the past for which he has never taken any medications. The patient is presently on no medications.

Two days ago, he started complaining of a dull chest ache that appeared to radiate to his left arm and lasted for a few minutes. He was brought to the emergency department and was noted to have an acute inferior myocardial infarction with complete heart block. I was consulted to evaluate the patient and proceeded with administration of TPA therapy and IV Atropine for complete heart block. At the present time the patient is in sinus rhythm and is presently receiving IV TPA. He denies any melena, hematochezia. Denies any shortness of breath, PND, orthopnea.

PAST MEDICAL HISTORY: He denies any history of hypertension or diabetes. He has a history of high cholesterol. He states that he had his cholesterol checked approximately 3 months ago and it was around 310. He used to smoke tobacco, one pack a day for 20 years. He quit smoking 6 months ago. He denies any history of coronary artery disease, myocardial infarction, or cerebrovascular accident.

He has a history of heart palpitations for which he is not taking any medications. He has never had an evaluation.

He has a history of kidney stones 2 years ago. He denies any history of peptic ulcer disease. He has a history of hemorrhoidal bleeding in the past. The last episode of bleeding was 6 or 7 months ago.

The patient denies any trauma or recent surgery.

ALLERGIES: Patient has no known drug allergies.

CHRONIC MEDICATIONS: None

SOCIAL HISTORY: He quit tobacco 6 months ago and denies alcohol abuse. He is a construction worker.

REVIEW OF SYSTEMS: Denies melena, hematochezia, hematemesis and he denies change in weight.

PHYSICAL EXAMINATION: This is a pleasant gentleman who appears slightly diaphoretic and is expressing having mild chest pain which is better from admission. He is presently receiving IV TPA. Vital signs are as follows: Blood pressure is 100/70; heart rate in the 80s. The neck shows no JVD, no carotid bruits. The lungs are clear and heart is regular rate with S4 gallop rhythm and no murmurs. The abdomen is soft and nontender. Extremities show no edema. The pulses of his femoral and dorsalis pedis are 2+ bilaterally. Neurological examination reveals an alert and oriented male ×3.

LABORATORY DATA: SMA-7, sodium 138, potassium 3.7, BUN 7, creatinine 0.9. CBC showed a white blood cell count of 12. Hematocrit 37, hemoglobin 13. Platelet count is 312. His EKG showed complete heart block with significant ST elevation in the inferior leads with reciprocal changes in the anteroseptal leads, consistent with an acute inferior wall myocardial infarction. His chest x-ray is pending.

Exam 1 Case Studies

HISTORY AND PHYSICAL EXAMINATION—PATIENT 8 (continued)

IMPRESSION AND PLAN: Acute myocardial infarction that appears to have started around 10:30 in the morning. He presented very early to the emergency department and was treated aggressively with intravenous TPA, intravenous aspirin, intravenous nitroglycerin.

We will continue the TPA and begin lidocaine. We will obtain cardiac enzymes and admit to CCU. The patient will need cardiac catheterization evaluated within 48 hours. If symptoms recur or patient does not have evidence of reperfusion will need urgent cardiac catheterization. If heart block occurs, will treat with intravenous Atropine on a p.r.n. basis. We will check a cholesterol and lipid profile in the hospital.

CONSULTATION—PATIENT 8

DATE: 4/20

CHIEF COMPLAINT: Vomiting blood

REVIEW OF SYSTEMS: This 45-year-old white male was seen in consultation because of GI bleeding. The patient was admitted one day ago with acute myocardial infarction. He was treated with TPA and later went to cardiac catheterization where he was found to have a lesion of the mid RCA and distal RCA. Today the patient exhibited hematemesis with retching. He has no past history of ulcer disease or GI bleeding.

PHYSICAL EXAMINATION: Physical examination reveals an adult male lying in bed. Blood pressure is 120/80, pulses 60. HEENT: Pale. LUNGS: Clear. HEART: Regular rate and rhythm.

ABDOMEN: Benign.

LABORATORY: WBC is 12, hemoglobin 12, and hematocrit 37

IMPRESSION: Upper GI bleeding; rule out ulcer disease

RECOMMENDATION: We will perform an upper endoscopy to be performed today after informed consent is obtained. Further recommendations are to follow.

PROGRESS NOTES—PATIENT 8

DATE	NOTE
4/19	This is a 45-year-old white male with a history of increased cholesterol, no prior coronary artery disease, MI or CVA. He presented with acute ischemia and heart block. He was given peripheral IV TPA; 1–1½ hours after TPA he had severe chest pain with elevated ST inferior leads. He was treated emergently for urgent catheter and PTCA.
	Post catheter/stent
	Procedure: Left heart catheter, coronary angio, left ventricular angiography
	Results: Normal LCA, 99% mid-RCA and 70 stenosis distal RCA, successful stent PTCA to mid-RCA with excellent results.
4/20	Cardiac: Patient continues to have pain. Will prepare for CABG when patient stable from GI perspective.
	GI: The patient experienced vomiting with flecks of blood after the cardiac catheterization. In light of apparent acute blood loss anemia will check for peptic ulcer. Probable reaction to anesthetics.
	Endoscopy Note:
	Preop: Gastrointestinal bleeding
	Postop: Gastrointestinal bleeding, etiology unknown
	Procedure: EGD
	Complications: None
4/21	Patient is scheduled for the OR today. Bleeding stable.
	OP Note:
	Preop: Critical stenosis of the mid-RCA and distal RCA
	Postop: Same
	Operation: CABG ×2
	Complications: None
4/22	Patient recovering well. No chest pain or shortness of breath. The wound looks good. Will monitor acute blood loss anemia. The patient declines blood transfusion.
4/23	Chest clear, no chest pain, abdomen is soft with bowel sounds. Will transfer to the floor.
4/24	Wound healing well, patient OOB ambulating, no chest pain, lungs clear.
4/25	Will discharge today. Patient to follow up in 1 week.

Exam 1 Case Studies

PHYSICIAN'S ORDERS—PATIENT 8

DATE	ORDER
4/19	Admit to CCU
	DX: Acute MI
	Cardiac enzymes q. 8 hours ×3
	CBC q. day ×3
	Meds:
	IV nitro @ 20 mg/min
	ASA 325 mg PO q. day
	Ticlid 250 mg PO b.i.d.
	Xanax 0.25 mg PO t.i.d. p.r.n.
	Restoril 30 mgs PO q. h p.r.n. for sleep
	Zantac 150 mg PO b.i.d.
	Daily PT and INR, PTT
	Diet: cardiac
	Vital signs q. 15 min ×8 then q.i.d.
	Bed rest
	O_2 at 2 L/min
	NS at 150 cc/hr for 10 hours
4/20	Lopressor 25 mg PO t.i.d.
	Social worker consult re: payment issues
	CBC at 6 p.m.
	NPO for now
	Possible endoscopy
	Postendoscopy orders
	Watch VS
	Resume previous orders
	No heparin or TPA
	Hgb and Hct q. 6 h
	NS at 125 cc/hr
	D/C ASA, Ticlid for now
	Tagamet drip per protocol
4/21	Postop CABG orders:
	Continue present ventilator settings
	Daily electrolytes and CBC
	Morphine sulfate 15 mg PO q. 4h p.r.n.
	TED stockings
	Weigh patient daily
	Routine weaning in a.m.
	Lidocaine 3 g/min
	Continue Tagamet drip

PHYSICIAN'S ORDERS—PATIENT 8 (*continued*)

4/22	Decrease Lidocaine to 2 g/min
	Extubate patient as soon as weaned from ventilator
	Chest tubes to low suction
	Oxygen face mask 4 L/min
	Encourage incentive spirometry
4/23	Nutrition consult re: low-fat, low-salt diet
	D/C Tagamet drip to 250 mg q. 6
	Benadryl p.r.n. for sleep
	Consult cardiac rehab
4/24	D/C oxygen
	Consult home healthcare for postsurgical monitoring
4/25	Discharge patient

OPERATIVE REPORT—PATIENT 8

DATE: 4/21

PREOPERATIVE DIAGNOSIS: Critical stenosis of mid right coronary artery and distal right coronary artery

POSTOPERATIVE DIAGNOSIS: Same

OPERATION: Coronary bypass ×2 using saphenous vein from aorta to right mid coronary artery and distal right coronary artery

ANESTHESIA: General

Under general anesthesia with arterial and pulmonary artery monitoring with sterile prep and drape, a sterile midline sternotomy was performed. The pericardium was opened. Purse-string sutures were placed in the ascending aorta and the right atrium. Extracorporeal circulation was undertaken at this point. The left greater saphenous vein was harvested from the right leg endoscopically. The patient was then placed on cardiopulmonary bypass. Cardioplegia was affected. The right coronary artery was dissected. Using a 6-0 Prolene suture an end-to-side anastomosis was created between the right mid coronary artery and the aorta. A second opening for end to side anastomosis was performed from the aorta to the distal right coronary artery. Following spontaneous contraction of the heart the patient was removed from cardiopulmonary bypass. Approximating the pericardium then began closure. Hemostasis was obtained. The sternum was approximated with a parasternal wire and fascia and skin with Vicryl. The patient tolerated the procedure well and was transferred to the recovery room in stable condition.

ENDOSCOPY REPORT—PATIENT 8

DATE: 4/20

Pre-gastrointestinal bleeding; rule out ulcers

Post-upper gastrointestinal bleeding; stomach and duodenum appear unremarkable

MEDS:

Demerol 50 mg IV

Versed 3 mg IV

PROCEDURE: Esophagogastroduodenoscopy

The patient was sedated and the scope inserted into the hypopharynx. There was fresh blood oozing from an area in the hiatal hernia pouch just below the gastroesophageal junction. The scope was passed farther down to visualize the remainder of the stomach and the duodenum. All areas appeared unremarkable with no other ulcers or lesions identified. The patient tolerated the procedure well. He did have some retching and vomiting after the scope was removed.

CARDIAC CATHETERIZATION SUMMARY—PATIENT 8

DATE: 4/19

PROCEDURE:

Left heart catheterization

Left ventricular angiography

Coronary angiography

Stent to mid right coronary artery

After obtaining informed consent the patient was taken to the cardiac catheterization laboratory. He was prepped and draped in the usual fashion and 2% Xylocaine was used to anesthetize the right groin. 6-French sheaths were introduced into the right femoral artery and vein and a 6-French multipurpose catheter was used for left heart catheterization, coronary angiography and left ventricular angiography using fluoroscopy and Omnipaque low osmolar contrast. I then proceeded to perform a Stent/PTCA to the mid RCA. An HTF wire was used to cross the RCA stenosis and a 4.0-mm J&J Stent was placed in the mid right coronary artery with excellent results. The final angiogram was obtained and the guiding catheterization was removed. The sheaths were securely sutured and the patient tolerated the procedure well without complications.

FINDINGS:

1. Left heart catheterization revealed an elevated resting left ventricular end-diastolic pressure of 18 mm Hg.

2. Left ventricular angiography revealed mild to moderate inferior wall hypokinesis with overall mildly depressed left ventricular systolic function and an estimated global ejection fraction of 45%.

3. Coronary angiography (using single catheter): The left coronary artery arises normally from the left sinus of Valsalva. The left main artery, left anterior descending coronary artery and its branches, and the circumflex artery and its branches have minimal irregularities.

The right coronary artery arises normally from the right sinus of Valsalva. There is a 99% very eccentric stenosis in the large mid right coronary artery and a 70% stenosis of the distal right coronary artery.

IMPRESSION: Arteriosclerotic coronary artery disease was found. There was a successful implantation of 4.0-mm J&J stent in the mid right coronary artery. This site was predilated with a 4.0-mm balloon, then followed by the insertion of a stent.

The mid right coronary artery shows excellent results. Pending the patient's progress we may have to proceed with CABG. The patient will remain on aspirin, Coumadin, and nitrates in the hospital. He will remain on intravenous heparin while his PT levels are adjusted.

LABORATORY REPORTS—PATIENT 8

HEMATOLOGY

DATE: 4/19

Specimen	Results	Normal Values
WBC	9.3	4.3–11.0
RBC	4.4 L	4.5–5.9
HGB	12.7 L	13.5–17.5
HCT	41	41–52
MCV	89	80–100
MCHC	33.9	31–57
PLT	Adequate	150–450

HEMATOLOGY—PATIENT 8

DATE: 4/20

Specimen	Results	Normal Values
WBC	7.7	4.3–11.0
RBC	4.4 L	4.5–5.9
HGB	12.0 L	13.5–17.5
HCT	41	41–52
MCV	89.6	80–100
MCHC	33.9	31–57
PLT	Adequate	150–450

HEMATOLOGY—PATIENT 8

DATE: 4/21

Specimen	Results	Normal Values
WBC	8.0	4.3–11.0
RBC	2.88 L	4.5–5.9
HGB	8.6 L	13.5–17.5
HCT	25.8 L	41–52
MCV	89	80–100
MCHC	33.9	31–57
PLT	Adequate	150–450

LABORATORY REPORTS—PATIENT 8 (continued)

HEMATOLOGY—PATIENT 8

DATE: 4/21

Specimen	Results	Normal Values
WBC	8.0	4.3–11.0
RBC	4.5	4.5–5.9
HGB	9.0 L	13.5–17.5
HCT	26.5 L	41–52
MCV	89	80–100
MCHC	33.9	31–57
PLT	Adequate	150–450

HEMATOLOGY—PATIENT 8

DATE: 4/21

Specimen	Results	Normal Values
WBC	8.0	4.3–11.0
RBC	4.5	4.5–5.9
HGB	9.3 L	13.5–17.5
HCT	27.3 L	41–52
MCV	89	80–100
MCHC	33.9	31–57
PLT	Adequate	150–450

HEMATOLOGY—PATIENT 8

DATE: 4/22

Specimen	Results	Normal Values
WBC	7.0	4.3–11.0
RBC	2.95 L	4.5–5.9
HGB	9.0 L	13.5–17.5
HCT	26.3 L	41–52
MCV	89	80–100
MCHC	33.9	31–57
PLT	Adequate	150–450

LABORATORY REPORTS—PATIENT 8 (continued)

HEMATOLOGY—PATIENT 8

DATE: 4/23

Specimen	Results	Normal Values
WBC	6.7	4.3–11.0
RBC	2.78 L	4.5–5.9
HGB	8.4 L	13.5–17.5
HCT	24.8 L	41–52
MCV	89.2	80–100
MCHC	34	31–57
PLT	Adequate	150–450

HEMATOLOGY—PATIENT 8

DATE: 4/24

Specimen	Results	Normal Values
WBC	8.0	4.3–11.0
RBC	4.3 L	4.5–5.9
HGB	9.2 L	13.5–17.5
HCT	27.0 L	41–52
MCV	89	80–100
MCHC	33.9	31–57
PLT	Adequate	150–450

HEMATOLOGY—PATIENT 8

DATE: 4/25

Specimen	Results	Normal Values
WBC	8.0	4.3–11.0
RBC	4.5	4.5–5.9
HGB	11.1 L	13.5–17.5
HCT	32 L	41–52
MCV	89	80–100
MCHC	33.9	31–57
PLT	Adequate	150–450

LABORATORY REPORTS—PATIENT 8 (*continued*)

CHEMISTRY—PATIENT 8

DATE: 4/19

Specimen	Results	Normal Values
GLUC	97	70–110
BUN	12	8–25
CREAT	1.0	0.5–1.5
NA	134 L	136–146
K	4.0	3.5–5.5
CL	109	95–110
CO_2	33 H	24–32
CA	9.1	8.4–10.5
PHOS	3.0	2.5–4.4
MG	2.0	1.6–3.0
CK	1,702 H	38–120
LD	327 H	106–270
CK MB	93.7 H	0.0–3.0
Relative Index	5.5	
AST	36	0–40
ALT	44	30–65
GCT	70	15–85
LD	110	100–190
ALK PHOS	114	50–136
URIC ACID	6.0	2.2–7.7
CHOL	275 H	0–200
TRIG	140	10–160

LABORATORY REPORTS — PATIENT 8 (continued)

CHEMISTRY—PATIENT 8

DATE: 4/20

Specimen	Results	Normal Values
GLUC	97	70–110
BUN	12	8–25
CREAT	1.0	0.5–1.5
NA	134 L	136–146
K	5.6 H	3.5–5.5
CL	109	95–110
CO_2	33 H	24–32
CA	9.1	8.4–10.5
PHOS	3.0	2.5–4.4
MG	2.0	1.6–3.0
CK	1,277 H	26–221
LD	345 H	106–210
CK MB	68.7 H	0.0–4.4
Relative Index	5.4	
AST	36	0–40
ALT	44	30–65
GCT	70	15–85
LD	110	100–190
ALK PHOS	114	50–136
URIC ACID	6.0	2.2–7.7
CHOL	275 H	0–200
TRIG	140	10–160

LABORATORY REPORTS—PATIENT 8 (continued)

CHEMISTRY—PATIENT 8

DATE: 4/21

Specimen	Results	Normal Values
GLUC	97	70–110
BUN	12	8–25
CREAT	1.0	0.5–1.5
NA	134 L	136–146
K	5.6 H	3.5–5.5
CL	109	95–110
CO_2	33 H	24–32
CA	9.1	8.4–10.5
PHOS	3.0	2.5–4.4
MG	2.0	1.6–3.0
CK	1024 H	26–221
LD	372 H	106–210
CK MB	40.3 H	0.0–4.4
Relative Index	3.9	
AST	36	0–40
ALT	44	30–65
GCT	70	15–85
LD	110	100–190
ALK PHOS	114	50–136
URIC ACID	6.0	2.2–7.7
CHOL	275 H	0–200
TRIG	140	10–160

RADIOLOGY REPORT—PATIENT 8

DATE: 4/19

CHEST, SUPINE: There is no gross evidence of acute inflammatory disease or congestive heart failure.

IMPRESSION: No acute disease

Exam 1 Case Studies

RADIOLOGY REPORT—PATIENT 8

DATE: 4/21

DIAGNOSIS: The patient appears to have undergone sternotomy. The heart appears normal. The endotracheal tube is in place as is the Swan-Ganz catheter.

IMPRESSION: Stable postoperative chest

EKG REPORT—PATIENT 8

DATE: 4/19

IMPRESSION: Elevated ST changes. Cannot eliminate the possibility of ischemia. Complete heart block is also noted.

EKG REPORT—PATIENT 8

DATE: 4/20

IMPRESSION: Acute inferior myocardial infarction. Complete heart block has resolved.

Choose the correct principal diagnosis code.

a. I21.01
b. I21.09
c. I21.19
d. I21.A1
e. I22.0

Choose the correct secondary diagnosis code(s).

- a. E78.2
- b. E78.5
- c. D62
- d. I25.10
- e. I44.2
- f. K92.0
- g. R11.2
- h. T41.205A
- i. Z87.891
- j. None apply

Choose the correct procedure code(s).

- a. 021009W
- b. 02703DZ
- c. 4A023N7
- d. B2111ZZ
- e. B2151ZZ
- f. 0DJ08ZZ
- g. 3E083GC
- h. 06BQ4ZZ
- i. 5A1221Z
- j. None apply

EMERGENCY DEPARTMENT RECORD—PATIENT 9

DATE OF ADMISSION: 10/24   **DATE OF DISCHARGE:** 10/24

HISTORY (EXPANDED PROBLEM FOCUSED): CHIEF COMPLAINT: RUQ abdominal pain.

HISTORY OF PRESENT ILLNESS: This 55-year-old African American male developed right upper quadrant abdominal pain after eating a greasy meal this evening.

PAST MEDICAL HISTORY: The patient is a one PPD smoker with COPD and OSA.

ALLERGIES: NKA

CHRONIC MEDICATIONS: Patient is oxygen dependent on 3 liters all the time.

REVIEW OF SYSTEMS: The patient describes the pain in the RUQ as a dull ache with onset after meal. Happened on one previous occasion about a week ago. Nothing appears to ease the pain. No fever, weight loss, diarrhea, or vomiting. Occasional nausea.

PHYSICAL EXAMINATION (EXPANDED PROBLEM FOCUSED):

GENERAL APPEARANCE: Appears to be a well-nourished 55-year-old black male in some discomfort. HEENT normal. Neck veins flat at 40-degree angle. No nodes felt in the neck, carotids, or groin. Carotid pulsations are normal. No bruits heard in the neck. Chest clear on percussion and auscultation. Heart is not enlarged. No thrills or murmurs. Rhythm is regular. BP 145/89. Liver and spleen not palpable. No masses felt in the abdomen. No ascites noted. No edema of the extremities. Pulses in the feet are good.

IMPRESSION: RUQ abdominal pain

PLAN: Zofran for nausea, x-ray of gallbladder

TREATMENT: Zofran administered orally. Venipuncture kit used to obtain blood draw for lab test. Gallbladder x-ray shows calculus in the gallbladder.

DISCHARGE DIAGNOSIS: Gallbladder calculus

INSTRUCTIONS ON DISCHARGE: Continue Zofran as needed for nausea. Schedule with Dr. Smith for outpatient cholecystectomy. Refrain from heavy, greasy meals.

Emergency Department E/M Level Evaluation and Management Mapping

The following are the acuity points needed to assign a particular level of CPT code:

Level 1 = 1–20

Level 2 = 21–35

Level 3 = 36–47

Level 4 = 48–60

Level 5 = > 61

Critical Care > 61 with constant physician attendance

CPT Codes Corresponding to Emergency Department E/M Level

Level 1 = 99281   99281–25 with procedure/laboratory/radiology

Level 2 = 99282   99282–25 with procedure/laboratory/radiology

Level 3 = 99283   99283–25 with procedure/laboratory/radiology

Level 4 = 99284   99284–25 with procedure/laboratory/radiology

Level 5 = 99285   99285–25 with procedure/laboratory/radiology

Emergency Department Acuity Points					
	5	10	15	20	25
Number of Meds Given	0–2	3–5	6–7	8–9	>10
Extent of Hx	Brief	PF	EPF	Detail	Comprehensive
Extent of Exam	Brief	PF	EPF	Detail	Comprehensive
Number of Tests Ordered	0–1	2–3	4–5	6–7	>8
Number of Supplies Used	1	2–3	4–5	6–7	>8

Choose the correct principal diagnosis code.

a. K80.10

b. K80.20

c. K80.21

d. R10.11

e. R10.13

Exam 1 Case Studies

Choose the correct secondary diagnosis code(s).

a. F17.200
b. F17.210
c. F17.290
d. G47.30
e. G47.33
f. J44.0
g. J44.1
h. J44.9
i. Z99.81
j. None apply

Choose the correct procedure code(s).

a. 99282
b. 99283
c. 99284
d. 99285
e. 99281-25
f. 99282-25
g. 99283-25
h. 99284-25
i. 99285-25
j. None apply

CCS

EXAM 2

Exam 2

A blank answer sheet for these multiple-choice questions can be found on page 161.

Domain 1 Coding Knowledge and Skills

1. A 55-year-old male was transferred to a nursing home for continuing care because of ventilator dependence following complications of cardiac bypass surgery. He was readmitted three weeks later due to ventilator associated pneumonia (VAP) due to *Pseudomonas aeruginosa*. How should the readmission be coded?

    a. T88.9XXA, J18.9, B96.5

    b. J16.8

    c. J95.851, B96.5

    d. J15.1, J95.851

2. Assign code(s) for the following diagnosis: Congestive heart failure due to hypertension.

I10	Essential (primary) hypertension
I11.0	Hypertensive heart disease with heart failure
I50.9	Heart failure, unspecified
I50.23	Acute on chronic systolic (congestive) heart failure

    a. I10, I50.9

    b. I11.0

    c. I50.23, I10

    d. I11.0, I50.9

3. A patient is seen for evaluation of a right orbital roof fracture. How should this be coded?

S02.121A	Fracture of orbital roof, right side, initial encounter for closed fracture
S02.31XA	Fracture of orbital floor, right side, initial encounter for closed fracture
S02.92XA	Unspecified fracture of facial bones, initial encounter for closed fracture
S02.91XA	Unspecified fracture of skull, initial encounter for closed fracture

    a. S02.121A

    b. S02.31XA

    c. S02.92XA

    d. S02.91XA

Domain 1

4. Patient presents in the ER with thrombosis of a loop PTFE hemodialysis fistula without mechanical complications. The physician performed a percutaneous thrombectomy of the left brachial vein. Assign a facility code for this outpatient procedure.

05CA3ZZ	Extirpation of matter from left brachial vein, percutaneous approach
36904	Percutaneous transluminal mechanical thrombectomy and/or infusion for thrombolysis, dialysis circuit, any method, including all imaging and radiological supervision and interpretation, diagnostic angiography, fluoroscopic guidance, catheter placement(s), and intraprocedural pharmacological thrombolytic injection(s)
36832	Revision, open, arteriovenous fistula; without thrombectomy, autogenous or nonautogenous dialysis graft (separate procedure)
37184	Primary percutaneous transluminal mechanical thrombectomy, noncoronary, arterial or arterial bypass graft, including fluoroscopic guidance and intraprocedural pharmacological thrombolytic injection(s); initial vessel

   a. 05CA3ZZ
   b. 36904
   c. 37184
   d. 36832

5. Patient admitted for laparoscopic repair of right diaphragmatic hernia. Assign the ICD-10-PCS procedure code for this surgery.

0BQT4ZZ	Repair diaphragm, percutaneous endoscopic approach
0BQT3ZZ	Repair diaphragm, percutaneous approach
0WQF4ZZ	Repair abdominal wall, percutaneous endoscopic approach
0BQT0ZZ	Repair diaphragm, open approach

   a. 0BQT4ZZ
   b. 0BQT3ZZ
   c. 0WQF4ZZ
   d. 0BQT0ZZ

6. A 45-year-old female patient comes in requesting an HIV test. The patient reports multiple male sexual partners recently. The patient undergoes HIV screening due to high-risk heterosexual behavior. What code(s) should be assigned?

   a. Z72.52, Z11.3
   b. Z11.4, Z72.51
   c. Z72.51, Z11.4
   d. Z11.3, Z72.52

7. A 23-year-old female is admitted for vaginal bleeding following a miscarriage two weeks prior to this admission. She is afebrile at this time and is treated with an aspiration dilation and curettage. Products of conception are found. Which of the following should be the principal diagnosis?

   a. O03.1, Delayed or excessive hemorrhage following incomplete spontaneous abortion
   b. O08.1, Delayed or excessive hemorrhage following ectopic and molar pregnancy
   c. O03.6, Delayed or excessive hemorrhage following complete or unspecified spontaneous abortion
   d. O07.1, Delayed or excessive hemorrhage following failed attempted termination of pregnancy

8. A patient presents to the emergency department with a fractured arm secondary to a fall precipitated by syncope and ataxia. The patient undergoes a closed reduction of the fracture in the emergency department and is then admitted for work up for metastatic carcinoma secondary to ataxia and syncope in a patient with recent history of lung cancer. The patient's work-up confirms recurrent lung carcinoma metastatic to the brain.

   The principal diagnosis should be:

   a. Fractured arm

   b. Syncope

   c. Metastatic carcinoma of the brain

   d. Carcinoma of the lung

9. A female patient with hematochezia presents to the hospital outpatient surgery department for a colonoscopy but the procedure was not performed due to elevated blood pressure. What is the first-listed diagnosis for this encounter?

   a. Elevated blood pressure

   b. Hematochezia

   c. Procedure not performed due to contraindication

   d. Procedure not performed for other reason

10. A patient was admitted for evaluation of chest pain. CAD was discovered upon completion of a left heart cath done with evaluation of the left heart, multiple coronary arteries, and aortography with low osmolar contrast. A non-drug eluting stent was required in the left anterior descending artery to alleviate the blockage. Prior to discharge the patient fell out of bed and suffered a left greater trochanter hip fracture. Open reduction, internal fixation was performed. Two days after the ORIF, the patient began running a fever and had chills. A post-op infection was diagnosed and a PICC line was inserted into the superior vena cava for administration of IV antibiotics over the next several weeks. Which of the following would be the principal procedure for this patient's stay?

    a. 02HV33Z

    b. 4A023N7

    c. 0QS704Z

    d. 02703DZ

11. A 55-year-old patient with AIDS admitted after being struck by car while walking in a parking lot. She has a comminuted, right femoral shaft fracture and a contusion of both hands and right elbow abrasion. The principal diagnosis should be the:

    a. AIDS

    b. Fractured femur

    c. Abrasion elbow

    d. Contusion hand

12. A patient takes Coumadin as prescribed and correctly administered. However, the patient develops hematuria secondary to the Coumadin use. The correct coding assignment for this case would be:

    a. Poisoning due to Coumadin

    b. Unspecified adverse reaction to Coumadin

    c. Hematuria, poisoning due to Coumadin

    d. Hematuria, adverse reaction to Coumadin

13. A patient with human immunodeficiency virus (HIV) with methicillin susceptible pneumonia due to *Staphylococcus aureus* was discharged from the acute-care setting. The physician documented that the pneumonia was HIV related. How should this be coded?

B20	Human immunodeficiency virus [HIV] disease
J15.20	Pneumonia due to staphylococcus, unspecified
J15.211	Pneumonia due to methicillin susceptible Staphylococcus aureus
J15.212	Pneumonia due to methicillin resistant Staphylococcus aureus
J17	Pneumonia in diseases classified elsewhere

   a. B20, J17

   b. J15.20, B20

   c. B20, J15.211

   d. J15.212, B20

14. A patient has a diabetic ulcer of the right foot. How should this patient's record be coded?

E11.40	Type 2 diabetes mellitus with diabetic neuropathy, unspecified
E11.621	Type 2 diabetes mellitus with foot ulcer
E11.69	Type 2 diabetes mellitus with other specified complication
L97.409	Non-pressure chronic ulcer of unspecified heel and midfoot with unspecified severity
L97.419	Non-pressure chronic ulcer of right heel and midfoot with unspecified severity

   a. E11.40, L97.419

   b. E11.40, L97.409

   c. E11.69, L97.419

   d. E11.621, L97.419

15. Acute peptic ulcer with perforation and hemorrhage and resulting blood loss anemia. What codes should be assigned?

K27.0	Acute peptic ulcer, site unspecified, with hemorrhage
K27.1	Acute peptic ulcer, site unspecified, with perforation
K27.2	Acute peptic ulcer, site unspecified, with both hemorrhage and perforation
D50.0	Iron deficiency anemia secondary to blood loss (chronic)
D62	Acute posthemorrhagic anemia

   a. K27.1, D62

   b. K27.0, D62

   c. K27.0, D50.0

   d. K27.2, D50.0

16. A patient is admitted as an inpatient and discharged with chest pain. After evaluation, it is suspected the patient may have gastroesophageal reflux disease (GERD). The final diagnosis was "Rule out GERD." The correct code assignment would be:

    a. Z03.89, Encounter for observation for other suspected diseases and conditions ruled out
    b. R10.11, Right upper quadrant pain
    c. K21.9, Gastroesophageal reflux disease without esophagitis
    d. R07.9, Chest pain, unspecified

17. If a patient undergoes an open biopsy for a frozen section immediately before the definitive surgery, how should this be coded with ICD-10-PCS codes?

    a. Definitive surgery only
    b. Open biopsy only
    c. Exploratory surgery
    d. Open biopsy and definitive surgery

18. The physician performed a bilateral myringotomy under general anesthesia for insertion of ventilating tubes on a 4-year-old male. This is due to chronic otitis media. What is the correct CPT code assignment and what modifier should be appended (if applicable) to this procedure code?

69421	Myringotomy including aspiration and/or Eustachian tube inflation requiring general anesthesia
69436	Tympanostomy (requiring insertion of ventilating tube), general anesthesia
–50	Bilateral procedure
–51	Multiple procedures
–RT	Right side
–LT	Left side

    a. 69421–RT, LT
    b. 69421–LT
    c. 69436–51
    d. 69436–50

19. A 59-year-old female patient presents with acquired hallux rigidus. Hallux rigidus repair is performed with resection of the joint with implant in the first left toe proximal phalanx. What codes would be assigned?

    a. M20.12, 28291–LT
    b. M20.22, 28291–TA
    c. M20.31, 28291–T5
    d. M20.12, 28291–TA

20. In outpatient surgery, a PTCA is completed with insertion of a drug-eluting stent in the left circumflex artery and a non-drug-eluting stent inserted into the left anterior descending artery of this 56-year-old female. Assign the correct CPT code(s) and modifier(s) for this procedure.

92920	Percutaneous transluminal coronary angioplasty; single major coronary artery or branch
+92921	each additional branch of a major coronary artery (List separately in additional to code for primary procedure.)
92928	Percutaneous transcatheter placement of intracoronary stent(s), with coronary angioplasty when performed; single major coronary artery or branch
+92929	each additional branch of a major coronary artery (List separately in addition to code for primary procedure.)
–LC	Left circumflex coronary artery
–LD	Left anterior descending coronary artery

a. 92921, 92920

b. 92928-LC, 92928-LD

c. 92920-LC, 92921-LD, 92928-LC, 92929-LD

d. 92921-LD, 92929-LD

21. Itching due to drug reaction to an antihistamine, properly taken. What are the appropriate codes and sequencing for this scenario?

L29.9	Pruritus, unspecified
R89.2	Abnormal level of other drugs, medicaments and biological substances in specimens from other organs, systems and tissues
T50.905A	Adverse effect of unspecified drugs, medicaments and biological substances, initial encounter
T45.0X1A	Poisoning by antiallergic and antiemetic drugs, accidental (unintentional), initial encounter
T45.0X5A	Adverse effect of antiallergic and antiemetic drugs, initial encounter

a. R89.2, T45.0X1A

b. R89.2, T45.0X5A

c. T50.905A, T45.0X1A

d. L29.9, T45.0X5A

22. A patient is admitted with abdominal pain. The discharge summary states "pancreatitis vs. noncalculus cholecystitis" as the final diagnoses. Both diagnoses are equally treated. Based on coding guidelines, what is the correct sequencing for these diagnoses?

a. Sequence either the pancreatitis or noncalculus cholecystitis first

b. Pancreatitis; noncalculus cholecystitis; abdominal pain

c. Noncalculus cholecystitis; pancreatitis

d. Sequence the abdominal pain first, followed by pancreatitis and noncalculus cholecystitis as secondary diagnoses

23. The "code, if applicable, any causal condition first" note in the ICD-10-CM Tabular List indicates that this code may be assigned when the causal condition is unknown or not applicable. When the causal condition is known, the code for that condition may be reported as which type of diagnosis?

    a. Comorbidity

    b. Manifestation

    c. Principal

    d. Qualified

24. A 70-year-old patient was admitted with pneumonia. The history and physical documented that the patient has a history of diabetes, hypertension, and migraine headache about 10 years ago without recurrence. The patient was administered IV antibiotics, metformin, and Altace during the hospitalization. What is the appropriate reporting and sequencing of these diagnoses?

    a. Diabetes, pneumonia, hypertension, and migraine headaches

    b. Pneumonia, diabetes, hypertension, and history of migraine headaches

    c. Pneumonia, diabetes, and hypertension

    d. Hypertension, diabetes, and pneumonia

25. Patient is admitted for removal of the gallbladder due to chronic cholecystitis. While performing a common bile duct exploration, a non-obstructive calculus was found and removed as well. Assign the correct coding sequence for a total laparoscopic cholecystectomy with percutaneous endoscopic removal of common bile duct stones.

    a. 0FC90ZZ, Extirpation of matter from common bile duct, open approach 0FB40ZZ, Excision of gallbladder, open approach

    b. 0FB40ZZ, Excision of gallbladder, open approach

    c. 0FC94ZZ, Extirpation of matter from common bile duct, percutaneous endoscopic approach 0FT40ZZ, Resection of gallbladder, open approach

    d. 0FT44ZZ, Resection of gallbladder, percutaneous endoscopic approach and 0FC94ZZ, Extirpation of matter from common bile duct, percutaneous endoscopic approach

26. A patient is admitted with hypotension due to dobutamine taken and prescribed correctly. How should this be coded and sequenced?

    a. T44.5X5A, Adverse effect of predominantly beta-adrenoreceptor agonists, initial encounter I95.1, Orthostatic hypotension

    b. I95.2, Hypotension due to drugs
       T44.5X5A, Adverse effect of predominantly beta-adrenoreceptor agonists, initial encounter

    c. T44.5X1A Poisoning by predominantly beta-adrenoreceptor agonists, initial encounter I95.89, Other hypotension

    d. T44.5X1A Poisoning by predominantly beta-adrenoreceptor agonists, initial encounter I95.81, Postprocedural hypotension

27. A female patient is diagnosed with congestive heart failure and also has a stage IV pressure ulcer. Which of the following POA indicators must be present so that the ulcer will be classified as an MCC for this admission?

    a. N

    b. Y

    c. W

    d. U

28. An inpatient undergoes a procedure and has a postoperative complication during the hospitalization. The insurance company will not pay for the entire amount requested. Which POA indicator is likely part of the reason for the reduced reimbursement?

   a. N
   b. Y
   c. W
   d. U

29. A patient with COPD is admitted with an acute exacerbation of chronic systolic heart failure. On day three of the admission, the provider documents the patient now is experiencing an acute exacerbation of his COPD. What is the POA indicator for the COPD exacerbation?

   a. Y
   b. N
   c. U
   d. W

30. A patient was admitted with hyperglycemia, uncontrolled thirst, constant hunger, and weight gain. Testing indicates that the patient has Type 2 diabetes which is noted in the discharge summary. What is the POA indicator for the diabetes?

   a. Y
   b. N
   c. U
   d. W

31. Which of the following is *not* a function of the outpatient code editor (OCE)?

   a. Editing the data on the claim for accuracy
   b. Specifying the action the FI should take when specific edits occur
   c. Assigning APCs to the claim (for hospital outpatient services)
   d. Determining payment-related conditions that require direct reference to ICD-10-CM codes

32. A patient has a laparoscopic appendectomy and this line item is showing on the bill:

CPT CODE	CPT DESCRIPTION	UNITS OF SERIVCE
44970	Laparoscopic Appendectomy	2

What coding edit would you expect based on this information?

   a. Medically Unlikely Edit
   b. Return to Provider Edit
   c. Medical Necessity Edit
   d. Procedure to Procedure Edit

33. A patient comes into the hospital with chest pain, shortness of breath, and a history of COPD. An MRI, chest x-ray, troponin, and CKMB are ordered. A coder might expect a medical necessity edit to be triggered for which test?

   a. Troponin
   b. Chest x-ray
   c. MRI
   d. CKMB

34. A coder assigns both 47562 and 47600 on the same patient's record. What coding edit should be triggered?

    a. Medical necessity

    b. Medically unlikely

    c. Sex/procedure edit

    d. Diagnosis/age edit

35. A Medicare patient admitted as an inpatient with acute abdominal pain is found to have appendicitis and has an appendectomy. The patient has a length of stay of two days. Reimbursement will be paid under which classification system?

    a. MS-DRG

    b. APG

    c. RBRVS

    d. APC

36. Medicare severity diagnostic-related groups (MS-DRGs) and ambulatory patient classifications (APCs) are dissimilar in that:

    a. There is only one MS-DRG per inpatient discharge but one or more APCs per outpatient visit

    b. There are many MS-DRGs per inpatient discharge but only one APC per outpatient visit

    c. There are more possible MS-DRGs for inpatients than there are APCs for outpatients

    d. There are up to three MS-DRGs per each inpatient discharge but there are up to seven APCs per outpatient visit

37. Which of the following services are paid under the outpatient prospective payment system (OPPS)?

    a. Ambulance services

    b. Same-day surgeries

    c. Physician fees

    d. Inpatient procedures

Use the following table to answer questions 38 and 39.

Admission Source Code	Admission Source Definition
1	Non-health care facility
2	Clinic
4	Transfer from Hospital
5	Transfer from Skilled or Intermediate Facility
6	Transfer from another Health Care Facility
7	Emergency Room
8	Court/Law Enforcement
E	Transfer from Ambulatory Surgery
F	Transfer from Hospice

38. A terminally ill patient under hospice care is admitted to Hospital A for palliative care. Two days later, the hospital must be evacuated due to an approaching hurricane and patients are transferred out. The terminally ill patient is transferred to another acute care facility, Hospital B. What is the correct admission source code for the admission to Hospital B?

   a. 1
   b. 4
   c. 6
   d. F

39. When a patient has had an outpatient cataract removal, and then requires admission, what is the appropriate admission source code that would be used?

   a. 2
   b. 4
   c. 7
   d. E

40. Elements of inpatient procedures that are typically abstracted by coders include which of the following?

   a. Procedure date and provider who performs procedure
   b. Provider who performs procedure and anesthetist
   c. Provider who performs procedure and any assistants
   d. Procedure date and CPT code

41. Which abstracted data elements can cause a potential increase in an MS-DRG assignment and corresponding increase in reimbursement?

   a. Race and payer
   b. Complications and comorbidities
   c. Ethnicity and age
   d. Discharge date and disposition

42. Which of the following data elements would a coding professional likely be responsible to abstract from a patient's record?

   a. Comorbidity
   b. Race
   c. Ethnicity
   d. Admission date

43. What factors of the APR-DRG system allow for capturing the extent of the patient's conditions and expected loss of life while an inpatient?

   a. Severity of illness and risk of mortality
   b. Severity of diagnosis and risk of morbidity
   c. Complications and comorbidities
   d. Hospital acquired conditions and present on admission

44. Which of the following diabetic conditions is considered an MCC?

   a. Type II diabetes without complication

   b. Type I diabetes without complication

   c. Type I diabetes with ketoacidosis

   d. Type II diabetes with polyneuropathy

45. Which of the following heart failure codes is considered an MCC?

   a. I50.9

   b. I50.43

   c. I50.32

   d. I50.20

46. Which of the following injuries would you expect to see with an MCC designation?

   a. Dislocation of jaw

   b. Laceration with foreign body of the neck

   c. Four-part humeral fracture of surgical neck

   d. Blister of the right eyelid and periocular area

Domain 2 Coding Documentation

47. A psychiatrist documents that a patient has wide mood swings ranging from excessive happiness to loss of energy and crying. What condition could be suggested by the psychiatrist's documentation?

   a. Bipolar disorder

   b. Major depression

   c. Anxiety

   d. Psychosis

48. A patient record has documentation of esophageal varices. Which condition, if related, would affect coding?

   a. Arthritis

   b. Liver disease

   c. Chronic obstructive pulmonary disease

   d. Erythema

49. A patient is admitted with lethargy, congestive heart failure, and pleural effusion. The patient underwent treatment with diuretics for the CHF, which has cleared. The pleural effusion required a thoracentesis to determine the cause. At the time of discharge, the effusion was decreased but not resolved. The correct coding assignment for this case would be:

   a. Congestive heart failure

   b. Pleural effusion

   c. Congestive heart failure and pleural effusion

   d. Lethargy, congestive heart failure, and pleural effusion

50. A 78-year-old patient is admitted with shortness of breath and a chest x-ray reveals infiltrates in the lung with pleural effusion. The patient also has a history of hypertension with left ventricular hypertrophy. The patient is given Lasix and the shortness of breath is relieved. From the information given, what is the probable principal diagnosis?

    a. Pneumonia
    b. Congestive heart failure
    c. Pleural effusion
    d. Chronic obstructive pulmonary disease

51. A patient was admitted directly from his primary physician's office due to suspected avian influenza. The admitting physician documentation indicated suspected avian influenza, along with signs and symptoms of avian influenza. The patient left against medical advice (AMA) before confirmatory lab tests could be drawn to identify the virus. The principal diagnosis should be coded from category:

    a. J09, Influenza due to certain identified influenza viruses
    b. J10, Influenza due to other identified influenza virus
    c. J11, Influenza due to unidentified influenza virus
    d. J12, Viral pneumonia, not elsewhere classified

52. In CPT, if a patient has two lacerations of the arm that are repaired; one 1.6 cm and the other 3.5 cm. What additional information does the coder need to assign the correct repair code?

    a. Specific location on the arm of each laceration
    b. If tissue adhesive was utilized
    c. The type of repair that was performed for each laceration
    d. If anesthesia was necessary for the procedure

53. The patient had an esophagoscopy to control a GI bleed. The coder would expect to see the following documentation in the chart for the diagnosis since upper gastrointestinal bleeding manifests as:

    a. Hematemesis
    b. Occult bleeding
    c. Melena
    d. Hematochezia

54. A patient was admitted with pneumonia. A sputum culture was able to identify *Mycoplasma pneumoniae* which the consulting pulmonologist documented as the cause of the pneumonia. The patient was also diagnosed with an *E. coli* UTI. In the final diagnosis statement, the attending physician documents *E. coli* pneumonia and UTI. How will the coder code the pneumonia?

    a. Assign the code based on the final diagnostic statement
    b. Assign the pneumonia code based on the consultant's documentation
    c. Assign the pneumonia code based on the sputum result
    d. Query the attending provider to clarify the pneumonia organism

55. A short-stay procedure H&P indicates a patient is coming for a left nephroureteral catheter exchange. The interventional radiologist performs the procedure and states that using the existing access, he places a guide wire into the kidney and removed the catheter. With the same access, over the guide wire the new nephroureteral catheter is inserted into the right kidney and ureter. What needs to be clarified in this scenario?

    a. Was the approach open or closed

    b. Was it done on the left or right

    c. Was this done percutaneously

    d. Was this procedure done under anesthesia

56. A patient has presented for back surgery with a diagnosis of lumbar stenosis. Documentation notes the patient has leg pain, tingling, and cramping as a result of the stenosis. In the patient's final diagnosis, the surgeon notes only lumbar stenosis. What other diagnosis appears to be missing from this statement based on the information provided?

    a. Neurogenic claudication

    b. Neuropathy

    c. Degenerative disc

    d. Spondylosis

57. When a patient is admitted and a discrepancy is noted in the documentation while the patient is still on the unit, who is responsible for obtaining clarity on the information?

    a. The charge nurse

    b. The clinical documentation specialist

    c. The coding professional

    d. The case manager

58. The following information was captured for a patient's ER visit: pulse 75, respirations 18, blood pressure 138/78, PERRLA, weight 267, height 60″, BMI 52. The patient complained of back pain after a fall. After no fractures were identified upon x-ray, the patient was discharged with a diagnosis of low back sprain as the only diagnosis. What diagnosis appears to be omitted in this scenario?

    a. Hypertension based on the elevated blood pressure reading

    b. Tachycardia based on the rapid pulse rate

    c. Morbid obesity based on the height, weight, and BMI

    d. Diplopia based on the PERRLA

Domain 3 Provider Queries

59. A patient has documentation on the discharge summary of urosepsis. The coding staff queries the attending physician about the condition and is provided further information that the patient has septicemia. This is in alignment with the laboratory tests and medication given, but the diagnosis of septicemia was not documented by the physician. How should the physician be requested to document the septicemia?

    a. A brand-new history and physical should be dictated to replace the one in the record.

    b. An addendum to the chart should be written.

    c. The new information should be squeezed in between lines within the progress notes of the last day.

    d. The query sheet will be sufficient to document this information.

60. A patient was admitted with Type 1 diabetes with proliferative diabetic retinopathy to have surgery for traction retinal detachment for macular edema. Which of the following questions would make a compliant query for this patient?

    a. Was the procedure performed on the left or right eye or bilateral eyes?

    b. Is the retinopathy a complication?

    c. Will you document use of insulin for this patient?

    d. Is there a comorbid condition that can be documented to increase the reimbursement?

61. Compliant multiple-choice queries:

    a. Must contain every possible option for the provider to choose from

    b. Can provide a new diagnosis with supporting clinical indicators

    c. Should provide a minimum of three options

    d. Are the preferred query format for establishing POA status

62. Which of the following is a noncompliant query format?

    a. Yes/no

    b. Open-ended

    c. Leading

    d. Multiple choice

63. Identify if the following query is compliant and the appropriate rationale.

    Dr. Jones, you state the patient has CHF in your discharge summary. Can you please indicate which type of the CHF the patient has?
    _____ Acute on chronic
    _____ Other

    a. Yes, this is compliant query as it is in multiple choice format and the requirement is to provide at least two choices.

    b. No, this is not a compliant query as it should have been an open-ended query format to allow the physician to identify the type of CHF.

    c. No, this is not a compliant query as this is leading the physician. More reasonable choices should have been provided.

    d. Yes, a multiple-choice query format is acceptable and referencing the diagnosed CHF makes this a compliant query.

64. A patient with a cephalic presentation anticipating a vaginal delivery failed to progress after a trial of oxytocin. Measurement of the fetal head was performed, and the patient was immediately taken to surgery for a cesarean section. What condition should the coder suspect and query the physician about?

    a. Twin pregnancy

    b. Early delivery

    c. Eclampsia

    d. Cephalopelvic disproportion

65. A 45-year-old woman underwent a carotid bypass and experienced a significant drop in blood pressure during the surgery. The documentation suggested the patient may have had a myocardial infarction. In accordance with coding guidelines, what should the coding professional do?

    a. Code complication of surgery NOS.

    b. Query the physician to determine if the patient had hypotension.

    c. Query the physician to determine if there was a complication of surgery.

    d. Code preoperative shock.

66. A patient's discharge summary does not contain a diagnosis that is documented by the anesthesiologist in a preoperative evaluation and that the diagnosis would impact MS-DRG assignment. The coder finds no evidence that the diagnosis contradicts documentation from the attending physician. The coder should:

    a. Code only from the discharge diagnoses

    b. Code the diagnosis reflected on the anesthesia preoperative evaluation

    c. Code the most severe symptom

    d. Query the attending physician regarding the clinical significance of that diagnosis

67. When an inpatient has had multiple tests to evaluate an abnormal finding but no definitive diagnosis has been documented, the coder should:

    a. Assign a code for the abnormal finding without confirming with the physician

    b. Not assign any code for the abnormal finding

    c. Assign a diagnosis code based on the coder's judgment

    d. Query the physician regarding whether a diagnosis should be assigned or not

68. A patient is admitted with Kaposi's sarcoma of the lung and a history of IV drug dependence is noted. Antiretroviral therapy is initiated for treatment with some alleviation of the patient's shortness of breath. Upon discharge, the only diagnosis listed was Kaposi's sarcoma of the lung. What other diagnosis might the coding professional expect to see with this condition and what action should be taken?

    a. CHF, add the code based on the "Code also" note in the Tabular for the sarcoma

    b. HIV, add the code based on the "Add additional code" note in the Tabular for the sarcoma

    c. CHF, query the physician based on the patient's shortness of breath and the "Code first" note in the Tabular for the sarcoma

    d. HIV, query the physician based on the previous drug dependence and the "Code first" note in the Tabular for the sarcoma

69. A patient is admitted to the hospital with a high fever, chills, tachycardia, and a respiration rate of 26. Lactic acidosis is noted in the labs. Pneumonia is diagnosed and the patient admitted to ICU where antibiotics are given along with Levophed to help maintain the patient's blood pressure which was in the extremely low range. The patient's breathing was erratic and mechanical ventilation was initiated. With a final diagnosis of pneumonia, what is the query opportunity for this record?

    a. Is this aspiration pneumonia?

    b. Is this septic shock?

    c. Is this *Staphylococcus aureus* pneumonia?

    d. Is this sepsis?

Domain 4 Regulatory Compliance

70. Two areas of documentation in the health record that are significant areas of focus of accrediting agencies are:

    a. Incident reports notation in the medical record and attorney's notes

    b. Past medical reports and social worker's notes

    c. Timeliness and legibility of medical documents

    d. Patient documentation and pastoral counseling

71. In facilities where electronic signatures are used for residents and attending physicians:

    a. Attending signature is all that is needed

    b. Resident signature is all that is needed

    c. Resident should cosign after the attending signs the documentation

    d. Attending should cosign after the resident signs the documentation

72. The coding supervisor is concerned that patients diagnosed with carcinoid colon tumors were miscoded as malignant during the last six months. To address this situation, what work processes could be undertaken?

    a. Obtain the cases of carcinoid colon tumors from the cancer registry, obtain the cases of malignant colon tumors from the billing system, import both lists into a spreadsheet, and compare them. The cases in the cancer registry but not coded as carcinoid in the billing system are likely malignant and should be manually reviewed.

    b. Compare the cases from the chart completion software with the billing software. Identify the cases that are not in the billing system. These cases should be manually reviewed to ensure they are not carcinoid tumors.

    c. Obtain the cases of malignant colon tumors from both the cancer registry and the billing system; import both lists into a spreadsheet and compare them. Identify the cases that are not in the tumor registry but are coded as malignant in the billing system. These cases should be manually reviewed to ensure they are not carcinoid tumors.

    d. Compare the cases from the transcription tracking software to the billing system. Identify the cases that are not in the transcription tracking software and are in the billing system. These cases should be manually reviewed to ensure they are not carcinoid tumors.

73. A patient undergoes an open reduction and internal fixation of a fractured femur. The record is coded with blood loss anemia because of a policy that specifies that this should be done when there is intraoperative blood loss of 500 cc or more documented in the operative report and the patient has low hemoglobin. Is this an ethical practice?

    a. It is ethical to code blood loss anemia because the policy requires it.

    b. It is ethical because the clinical signs are documented in the record.

    c. It is unethical because the patient must also have a blood transfusion in order for blood loss anemia to be coded.

    d. It is unethical because the physician did not document the blood loss anemia in the progress notes.

Exam 2

Use the information in the following table to answer questions 74 through 76.

Billing Number	Status Indicator	CPT/HCPCS	APC	Reimbursement*
989323	T	10060	0006	$500
989323	T	64605	0220	$1,000
989323	X	71045	0260	$50.00
989323	S	38230	0112	$2,000

*This is not the actual status indicator, APC number, or reimbursement for the designated APC.
**Status Indicators

S—Significant Procedure, Not Discounted when Multiple
T—Significant Procedure, Multiple Reduction Applies
X—Ancillary Services

74. The information in the table represents the APCs and associated data for all the CPT codes assigned for a patient's encounter. From the information provided, what would be the total reimbursement for this patient?

   a. $3,550
   b. $3,000
   c. $3,050
   d. $3,300

75. What percentage will the facility be paid for procedure code 10060?

   a. 50%
   b. 75%
   c. 0%
   d. 100%

76. If another status S procedure were performed, how much would the facility receive for the second status S procedure?

   a. 50%
   b. 75%
   c. 0%
   d. 100%

77. What is assigned to CPT codes to indicate whether a service or procedure will be separately reimbursed under the OPPS?

   a. Ambulatory payment classifications
   b. Payment status indicators
   c. Payment modifiers
   d. Diagnosis-related groups

78. The conditions that Medicare put on the hospital acquired conditions list are:

   a. Low volume
   b. Preventable
   c. High risk
   d. Surgical

79. Under which of the following circumstances does a facility lose a potential increase in reimbursement when a hospital acquired condition (HAC) is coded without a POA indicator of "Y"?

    a. When the HAC is the only CC/MCC on the account
    b. When the HAC is listed as the principal diagnosis
    c. When the HAC is coded along with a surgical procedure
    d. When the HAC is the only diagnosis listed

80. Hospital acquired conditions and the present on admission indicator are used to identify:

    a. Safety issues
    b. Quality issues
    c. Risk issues
    d. Documentation issues

81. Under HIPAA every organization must have:

    a. Privacy and Security Officers
    b. Security and Compliance Officers
    c. Compliance and Safety Officers
    d. Safety and Privacy Officers

82. A routine computer back-up procedure is an example of a security program that ensures data loss does not occur. This type of control is:

    a. Computer
    b. Validity
    c. Responsive
    d. Preventive

83. The patient was admitted for prostate carcinoma. This was treated with radiation. A member of the medical staff who was not associated with the patient's care requests to see the patient's record. What should the coder do?

    a. Provide the record to the physician.
    b. Report the incident to hospital security.
    c. Ask the physician to come back when the supervisor gets back.
    d. Explain that providing the record would violate the privacy policy.

84. In most circumstances, the person who authorizes release of medical information is:

    a. Chief executive officer
    b. Patient
    c. Physician
    d. Nurse

85. The combination of username and password is known what type of authentication?

    a. Context-based
    b. User-based
    c. Single-factor
    d. Two-factor

86. Which of the following are categories of standards under the HIPAA Security Rule?

    a. Administrative, technical, and physical
    b. Technical, physical, and governance
    c. Physical, governance, and administrative
    d. Governance, administrative, and technical

87. According to the AHIMA Standards of Ethical Coding, "A coder should protect the confidentiality of the health record at all times and refuse to access protected health information not required for coding-related activities." Which of the following is *not* considered a coding-related activity?

    a. Coding quality evaluation
    b. Review of records assigned each day
    c. Risk analysis of medical record documentation
    d. Completion of abstracting

88. A patient is admitted with vaginal bleeding. One of the concurrent coding analysts reviewing information in the chart has determined that there may be an additional procedure code but there is no operative report to provide definitive information. Coding the additional procedure as the documentation stands now would be considered an ethical practice if:

    a. The vice president of finance approves adding the code now
    b. The billing department wants this; it can be done
    c. Under no circumstances could this be done
    d. The coding supervisor approves coding the procedure

89. A coder is working from his work queue and gets assigned the outpatient surgery record of the hospital administrator. Is this an ethical issue? Why or why not?

    a. Yes, only the coding supervisor should code the record of the administrator
    b. Yes, the coder should never work on a chart of another hospital employee
    c. No, the coder can code the record as normal and look at previous encounters
    d. No, the coder can assign codes for the encounter without an ethical concern

90. An RHIT, who plans to sit for her RHIA certification in six months, wants to apply for the open director of medical records position at her organization. The job description states that the applicant must have an RHIA credential. Ethically, can the RHIT apply for the position?

    a. Yes, as long as she lists her RHIT credential on the application
    b. No, she does not have the required credential and should not apply
    c. No, if she lists the RHIA credential she will be lying
    d. Yes, since she plans to get the RHIA credential she can list it and apply

91. A coding supervisor performs an internal audit on the coding staff. The overall accuracy results are 85% and the expectation is 95%. She decides to eliminate the worst records from the audit in order to bolster the score which then becomes 93% and will make her look better to her boss. Is this ethically okay for her to do?

   a. Yes, internal audit criteria are determined by the coding supervisor and can be changed by her.
   b. Yes, if her boss approves of the elimination of the records, then it fine and there is no ethical issue.
   c. No, only the HIM Director can make changes to the audit including the number of records reviewed.
   d. No, the audit criteria should not be altered to provide a better score or improve the supervisor's status.

92. AHIMA's Standards of Ethical Coding apply to which of the setting(s) below?

   a. Acute inpatient
   b. Outpatient
   c. Provider offices
   d. All settings

93. An inpatient is discharged with a diagnosis of "either irritable bowel or pancreatitis." Which condition would be the principal diagnosis?

   a. Code both and sequence according to the circumstances of the admission
   b. Pancreatitis
   c. Irritable bowel syndrome
   d. Observation for suspected gastrointestinal condition

94. According to the UHDDS, the definition of a *secondary diagnosis* is a condition that:

   a. Is recorded in the patient record
   b. Receives evaluation and is documented by the physician
   c. Receives clinical evaluation, therapeutic treatment, further evaluation, extends the length of stay, increases nursing monitoring and care
   d. Is considered to be essential by the physicians involved and is reflected in the record

95. The best answer to describe how the UHDDS defines a comorbidity is a diagnosis that:

   a. Affects the payment rate
   b. Occurs after admission
   c. Is not documented
   d. Preexists before admission

96. A condition that is established after study to be chiefly responsible for the admission is the:

    a. Reason for visit
    b. Principal procedure
    c. A complication of outpatient care
    d. Principal diagnosis

97. The UHDDS definition of principal procedure indicates that the principal procedure can be assigned for which of the following?

    a. Addressing complications
    b. Exploration
    c. Diagnostic
    d. Clinical evaluation

Multiple Choice Exam 2 Answers

1.	26.	51.	76.
2.	27.	52.	77.
3.	28.	53.	78.
4.	29.	54.	79.
5.	30.	55.	80.
6.	31.	56.	81.
7.	32.	57.	82.
8.	33.	58.	83.
9.	34.	59.	84.
10.	35.	60.	85.
11.	36.	61.	86.
12.	37.	62.	87.
13.	38.	63.	88.
14.	39.	64.	89.
15.	40.	65.	90.
16.	41.	66.	91.
17.	42.	67.	92.
18.	43.	68.	93.
19.	44.	69.	94.
20.	45.	70.	95.
21.	46.	71.	96.
22.	47.	72.	97.
23.	48.	73.	
24.	49.	74.	
25.	50.	75.	

CCS

EXAM 2
CASE STUDIES

Note: Review the Guidelines for Coding the CCS Exam Preparation Case Studies in the Introduction of this book.

SAME-DAY SURGERY SUMMARY—PATIENT 1

DATE OF ADMISSION: 12/30 **DATE OF DISCHARGE:** 12/30

DISCHARGE DIAGNOSIS: Bunion of 1st metatarsal, left foot

ADMISSION HISTORY: This is a 45-year-old white female in good health. Her family physician has performed a history and physical that demonstrated her health is within normal limits. The patient has no known allergies, good pedal pulses. The patient has a bunion of the left 1st metatarsal.

COURSE IN HOSPITAL: The patient was admitted to same-day surgery for osteotomy of the 1st metatarsal. The patient was taken to the OR where this was accomplished. The patient tolerated the procedure well and is discharged to home in stable condition.

INSTRUCTIONS ON DISCHARGE:

Keep foot elevated.

Keep dressing dry; do not change until seen by your physician.

Use surgical shoe.

Take Percocet 2.5 mg every 4 hours as needed for pain.

HISTORY AND PHYSICAL EXAMINATION—PATIENT 1

DATE: 12/30

HISTORY OF PRESENT ILLNESS: The patient has had increased long-term pain with difficulty ambulating.

PAST MEDICAL HISTORY: The patient has no major health problems and has not undergone major surgery.

ALLERGIES: None known

CHRONIC MEDICATIONS: None

FAMILY HISTORY: Noncontributory

PHYSICAL EXAMINATION:

IMPRESSION: B.P. 130/88, pulse is 68, respirations 20, temp 97.3. HEENT, within normal limits. Heart, normal. Lungs, clear. Abdomen, soft with bowel sounds. Pelvic and rectal deferred. Extremities, normal except bunion on 1st metatarsal.

PLAN: Osteotomy with excision of 1st metatarsal eminence

PROGRESS NOTES—PATIENT 1

DATE	NOTE
12/30	This is a 45-year-old female admitted for osteotomy to relieve long-term pain in the left foot. The patient is good health.
	D/C when stable as per discharge criteria.
	Patient admitted for surgery.

OP-NOTE:

PREOP DX: Bunion of 1st metatarsal

POSTOP DX: Same

OPERATION: Osteotomy with excision of 1st metatarsal eminence

ANES: Digital

Good circulation and sensation. Will encourage patient to ambulate with splint and crutches.

Discharge when stable. Follow up in one week with my office.

DISCHARGE MEDICATIONS: Percocet 2.5 mg every 4 hours p.r.n. for pain

PHYSICIAN'S ORDERS—PATIENT 1

DATE	ORDER
12/30	Admit to Same-Day Surgery Unit
	Prep for surgery
	Vistaril 50 mg PO 1 hour preop
	Atropine 0.8 mg PO 1 hour preop
	Postop Orders:
	Continue to elevate foot.
	Percocet 2.5 mg every 4 hours p.r.n. for pain.
	Discharge patient when surgical shoe procured.

OPERATIVE REPORT—PATIENT 1

DATE: 12/30

PREOPERATIVE DIAGNOSIS: Bunion of the 1st metatarsal head, left foot

POSTOPERATIVE DIAGNOSIS: Same

OPERATION: Osteotomy with partial excision of the 1st left metatarsal head

ANESTHESIA: Digital

OPERATIVE PROCEDURE: With the patient under local standby anesthesia and in the supine position she was properly prepped and draped. The tourniquet was applied about the left ankle superior to the malleoli.

A lazy "S" type incision was made on the lateral side of the 1st metatarsal head. This incision was deepened by blunt and sharp dissection until the capsule of the 1st metatarsophalangeal joint, left was reached. A linear incision measuring approximately 4 cm in length was made. An osteotomy through the neck of the same bone was undertaken with an osteotome. Following alignment of bone, a wire link was placed. The joint capsule was closed with continuous suture of 2-0 chromic catgut and the subcutaneous tissue was closed with continuous suture of 4-0 chromic catgut and the skin was closed with continuous suture of 4-0 nylon.

The wound was dressed with Vaseline gauze and gentle fluff pressure dressing. The patient was discharged from the operating suite in good condition noting that vascularity had returned to all 5 toes.

PATHOLOGY REPORT—PATIENT 1

DATE: 12/30

SPECIMEN: Bunion from the 1st toe left foot

GROSS DESCRIPTION: The specimen consists of a dome-shaped fragment of hypertrophic osseous tissue that measures 1.2 × 1.1 × 0.5 cm. Decalcification.

MICROSCOPIC DESCRIPTION: Sections of the decalcified tissue reveal fragments of hypertrophic osteocartilaginous tissue. No evidence of metastatic disease or neutrophilic inflammatory infiltrate was noted.

DIAGNOSIS: Bone (left 1st toe): Fragments of hypertrophic osteocartilaginous tissue

Choose the correct principal diagnosis code.

a. M21.611
b. M21.612
c. M21.619
d. M21.621
e. M21.622

Choose the correct secondary diagnosis code(s).

a. E03.9
b. E11.9
c. E11.22
d. E78.2
e. E78.5
f. I10
g. M79.671
h. M79.672
i. M79.675
j. None apply

Choose the correct procedure code(s).

a. 28292-LT
b. 28292-TA
c. 28295-RT
d. 28295
e. 28296-LT
f. 28296-TA
g. 28297-T5
h. 28298-T5
i. 28299
j. 28299-RT

Exam 2 Case Studies

EMERGENCY DEPARTMENT RECORD—PATIENT 2

DATE OF ADMISSION: 8/19   **DATE OF DISCHARGE:** 8/19

HISTORY (PROBLEM FOCUSED):

ADMISSION HISTORY: This is a 13-year-old African-American male. He was short of breath, used his inhaler as prescribed but continued to have wheezing and shortness of breath.

ALLERGIES: None

CHRONIC MEDICATIONS: Albuterol inhaler

FAMILY HISTORY: Noncontributory

SOCIAL HISTORY: Noncontributory

REVIEW OF SYSTEMS: His integumentary, musculoskeletal, cardiovascular, genitourinary, and gastrointestinal systems are negative.

PHYSICAL EXAMINATION (EXTENDED PROBLEM FOCUSED):

GENERAL APPEARANCE: This is an alert, cooperative young male in acute distress.

HEENT: PERRLA, extraocular movements are full

NECK: Supple

CHEST: Lungs reveal wheezes and rales. Heart has normal sinus rhythm.

ABDOMEN: Soft and nontender, no organomegaly

EXTREMITIES: Examination is normal.

LABORATORY DATA: Urinalysis is normal, EKG normal, chest x-ray is normal. CBC and diff show no abnormalities.

IMPRESSION: Moderately persistent asthma with exacerbation

PLAN: Administer IM epinephrine and intravenous theophylline

TREATMENT: Following IM administration of epinephrine and IV theophylline which ran for 47 minutes, the patient's asthma abated. One venipuncture set and one IV set were used to administer the medication over 30 minutes.

DISCHARGE DIAGNOSIS: Asthma, moderately persistent with exacerbation

DISCHARGE INSTRUCTIONS: The patient was instructed to take his prescribed medications as directed by his primary care physician and to return to the ER if he had any further asthma.

Emergency Department Evaluation and Management (E/M) Mapping

Code the procedures that are done in the emergency department as well as the facility E/M code derived from the point values, CPT codes and table below.

Emergency Department E/M Level Point Value Key

Level 1 = 1–20
Level 2 = 21–35
Level 3 = 36–47
Level 4 = 48–60
Level 5 = > 61
Critical Care > 61 with constant physician attendance

CPT Codes Corresponding to Emergency Department E/M Level

Level 1	99281	99281–25 with procedure/laboratory/radiology
Level 2	99282	99282–25 with procedure/laboratory/radiology
Level 3	99283	99283–25 with procedure/laboratory/radiology
Level 4	99284	99284–25 with procedure/laboratory/radiology
Level 5	99285	99285–25 with procedure/laboratory/radiology

Emergency Department Acuity Points					
	5	10	15	20	25
Number of Meds Given	1–2	3–5	6–7	8–9	≥10
Extent of Hx	Brief	PF	EPF	Detail	Comprehensive
Extent of Examination	Brief	PF	EPF	Detail	Comprehensive
Number of Tests Ordered	0–1	2–3	4–5	6–7	≥8
Number of Supplies Used	1	2–3	4–5	6–7	≥8

Choose the correct principal diagnosis code.

a. J45.21
b. J45.32
c. J45.40
d. J45.41
e. J45.52

Choose the correct secondary diagnosis code(s).

a. E86.0
b. I10
c. J45.31
d. K21.9
e. R06.02
f. R06.2
g. R06.89
h. R50.9
i. R51
j. None apply

Choose the correct procedure code(s).

a. 99282-27
b. 99283-24
c. 99284-25
d. 99285-24
e. 96365
f. 96366
g. 96367
h. 96372-59
i. 96374
j. 96375-59

SAME-DAY PROCEDURE—PATIENT 3

INDICATIONS: CAD

PROCDURES PERFORMED: Left heart catheterization, left ventriculography, coronary angiography, drug-eluting stent to left anterior descending coronary artery

PROCEDURE: After obtaining informed consent the patient was taken to the cardiac catheterization laboratory. He was prepped and draped in the usual fashion and 2% Xylocaine was used to anesthetize the right groin. 6-French sheaths were introduced into the right femoral artery and vein and a 6-French multipurpose catheter was used for left heart catheterization, coronary angiography, and left ventricular angiography. I then proceeded to perform a PTCA with a stent of the LAD. A HTF wire was used to cross the LAD stenosis and a balloon catheter inserted and inflated for pre stent dilation.
A 4.0 mm Cypher stent was placed in the left anterior descending coronary artery and the stent deployed by additional balloon angioplasty. Excellent results were obtained. The final angiogram was obtained and the guiding catheter was removed. The sheaths were securely sutured and the patient tolerated the procedure well without complications.

FINDINGS:

Left heart catheterization revealed an elevated resting left ventricular end diastolic pressure of 18 mm Hg.

Left ventriculography: Viewed in the RAO projection with normal systolic wall motion. The end-diastolic pressure is 18 to 20 mm Hg. There is no gradient detected.

Coronary angiography (using single catheter): The right coronary vessel has dominant structure with minor luminal irregularities only. The left main is normal with the left anterior descending coronary artery having a 95% stenosis and the circumflex marginal system with a 10% to 20% plaquing only.

LAD stent underlying: Left anterior descending coronary vessel was easily isolated and the primary stent intervention was carried out with a 3.0 Cypher drug-eluting stent. Final sizing was 3.1 mm resulting in 0% residual stenosis and maintenance of TIMI III flow distally in the LAD system.

CONCLUSION: Critical single-vessel obstructive coronary artery disease involving the LAD successfully treated with drug-eluting stent technology. The left anterior descending coronary artery shows excellent results. Preserved left ventricular systolic wall motion.

Exam 2 Case Studies

Choose the correct principal diagnosis code.

   a. I25.10
   b. I25.119
   c. I25.720
   d. I25.758
   e. I25.761

Choose the correct secondary diagnosis code(s).

   a. E11.22
   b. I10
   c. I21.A1
   d. I25.119
   e. I50.32
   f. I73.9
   g. N18.6
   h. N39.0
   i. R33.9
   j. None apply

Choose the correct procedure code(s).

   a. 92920-RC
   b. 92921
   c. 92924-RC
   d. 92925
   e. 92928-LD
   f. 92929
   g. 92933-LD
   h. 93458
   i. 93459
   j. 93460

PAIN MANAGEMENT—PATIENT 4

DATE: 1/20XX

CHIEF COMPLAINT: Weakness, pain, vomiting, sleepiness

HISTORY OF PRESENT ILLNESS:

The patient is a 55-year-old female who presents to the same-day surgery department with her family. The patient has anal cancer metastatic to the kidney-lung-brain areas. She has been seen here multiple times for management of her pain. She has been having increasing weakness and vomiting at home, decreased mentation. She has been bedridden for at least the last 4 weeks.

REVIEW OF SYSTEMS:

She has occasional headaches and seizures. Back and chest pain. No syncope, cough, or shortness of breath. She has had repeated bouts of nausea and vomiting, no obvious urinary frequency, urgency, or dysuria. She has had decreased mentation. The review of systems is otherwise negative.

PAST MEDICAL HISTORY:

ILLNESSES:

1. Cancer as above
2. History of hypertension
3. She has seizures secondary to brain metastases

MEDICATIONS:

Per list include

1. Dilantin 300 mg p.o. b.i.d.
2. Lantus insulin
3. Dexamethasone
4. Protonix
5. Xanax
6. Atenolol
7. Norvasc
8. Reglan
9. Benadryl
10. Antivert
11. Zyvox
12. Depakote
13. Lorazepam

PAIN MANAGEMENT—PATIENT 4 (*continued*)

ALLERGIES:

1. Levaquin
2. Penicillin

The patient lives at home. She is a nonsmoker. She is here with multiple family members. She is married.

PHYSICAL EXAMINATION:

VITAL SIGNS: Temperature 98.7 degrees, pulse 72, respiratory rate 16, blood pressure 142/91

GENERAL: This is an ill-appearing female with decreased mentation and speech.

HEENT: PERRLA

NECK: Supple

CHEST: Breath sounds are equal bilaterally. Clear. No wheezes, rales, or rhonchi.

CARDIOVASCULAR: No obvious murmurs, gallops or rubs.

ABDOMEN: Soft. No specific tenderness, guarding, rebound.

EXTREMITIES: Joints have full range of motion.

MUSCULOSKETAL: Pain in lower back and chest.

NEUROLOGIC: Moves all extremities well.

SKIN: Normal skin. No acute rashes or lesions.

DIAGNOSES: Pain due to metastatic anal cancer.

Upon admission to the same-day surgery unit an IV was started. She was given 500 cc normal saline. I have updated the family and written orders. I have also reviewed her records, especially her previous labs, as well as her history of metastatic cancer.

RADIOLOGY:

CLINICAL HISTORY: Metastatic anal cancer

DESCRIPTION OF EXAM: Ultrasound and fluoroscopic guided PICC line insertion

RESULT: The patient's left arm was prepped and draped in the usual sterile fashion. A tourniquet was applied in the axilla. The skin was infiltrated with 1% lidocaine for local anesthesia. Using real time ultrasound guidance, a 21-gauge micropuncture needle was introduced into the left brachial vein. The needle was exchanged over an 0.018 microvena guide wire for a 5 French peel-away sheath. The introducer and guidewire were removed. A 5 French dual lumen PICC line was then advanced over the microvena guidewire and positioned with the tip at the superior vena cava/right atrial junction. Each lumen was aspirated and flushed with saline. The line was heparinized. The line was secured to the patient's skin. A sterile dressing was applied. The patient tolerated the procedure well. There were no immediate complications.

CONCLUSION: Ultrasound and fluoroscopic guided PICC line insertion performed. Dual lumen 5 French PICC line inserted in the left brachial vein with the tip at the superior vena cava or right atrial junction.

Choose the correct principal diagnosis code.

   a. G89.0
   b. G89.18
   c. G89.3
   d. G89.4
   e. R52

Choose the correct secondary diagnosis code(s).

   a. C19
   b. C20
   c. C21.0
   d. C78.00
   e. C79.00
   f. C79.31
   g. I10
   h. K21.9
   i. R56.9
   j. None apply

Choose the correct procedure code(s) that apply.

   a. 36557
   b. 36558
   c. 36560
   d. 36561
   e. 36563
   f. 36565
   g. 36566
   h. 36569
   i. 36572
   j. 36573

SAME-DAY SURGERY—PATIENT 5

DISCHARGE DIAGNOSIS: Severe infection on the right foot

CHIEF COMPLAINT: Infection on the right foot

HISTORY OF PRESENT ILLNESS:

This 82-year-old white female reports that she has bilateral lower extremity neuropathy of unknown etiology and she has been worked up extensively in the past by neurology and is currently being treated with Neurontin for her lower extremity discomfort. She reports that she rarely goes barefoot, but she has been in the last 2 weeks in the process of moving into a new apartment. She did walk barefoot for a time period across her new Berber carpet and noted the next morning to have sustained some blisters on the bottoms of her feet. Despite caring for them conservatively at home, they proceeded to become infected and she was seen in the office by Dr.'s nurse practitioner. At that time she also had a urinary tract infection and therefore she was put on p.o. Levaquin to cover both problems. She reports that her left foot improved dramatically, but the right foot continued to worsen to the point where she was unable to bear weight on it and so is admitted to the same-day surgery today.

PAST MEDICAL HISTORY:

ILLNESSES:

1. Hypertension
2. Peripheral neuropathy
3. Hypothyroidism

SURGERIES:

1. Appendectomy
2. Cholecystectomy

ALLERGIES: Sulfur

MEDICATIONS:

1. Atenolol 50 mg daily
2. Maxzide 50/75 mg 1 p.o. q.d.
3. Synthroid 25 mcg 1 p.o. q.d.
4. Quinine
5. Calcium plus vitamin D
6. Benadryl
7. Tylenol
8. Vitamin C
9. Vitamin E
10. Multivitamin
11. Percocet 2.5 mg p.r.n.
12. Neurontin 300 mg 1 p.o. t.i.d.

SAME-DAY SURGERY—PATIENT 5 (*continued*)

SOCIAL HISTORY:

The patient lives independently. She is currently moving into an apartment. She states that her husband is alive, but a resident of a nursing home and she is currently moving to be closer to him. She denies tobacco or alcohol use. The patient is married. She does not smoke. She is retired. She lives at home.

REVIEW OF SYSTEMS: Is as above

FAMILY HISTORY: Noncontributory

PHYSICAL EXAMINATION:

- **GENERAL:** Reveals a well-developed, well-nourished, elderly female in no apparent distress.
- **VITAL SIGNS:** Temperature 96.8 degrees, pulse 12, respirations 18, blood pressure 141/76, oxygen saturation 100% on room air
- **HEENT:** Benign
- **NECK:** Supple without lymphadenopathy
- **LUNGS:** Clear to auscultation bilaterally
- **CV:** Regular rate and rhythm without murmur, rub, or gallop
- **ABDOMEN:** Soft, nontender, nondistended. Normal bowel sounds.

EXTREMITIES: Bilateral lower extremities with 1 plus pitting edema bilaterally. The right foot has evidence of previous insult the first MTP joint with minimal redness, tenderness, and peeling skin from a previous blister. The right lower extremity in the area of the 1st MTP joint is swollen. The foot is somewhat warm to touch and the patient denies pain.

DIAGNOSTIC DATA: Plain x-ray was reported as negative for bone or joint involvement though it does show the soft tissue swelling. Basic metabolic profile was within normal limits with hemoglobin 10.9. CBC showed a white count that was not elevated. X-ray of the foot showed no osteomyelitis.

ASSESSMENT AND PLAN:

1. Abscess of the foot in the area of the right 1st metatarsophalangeal (MTP) joint and the patient is admitted for incision and drainage and debridement.
2. Hypertension. Seems controlled. Will continue her home medications.
3. Hypothyroidism. Controlled. Continue home medications and check a TSH.

PROGRESS NOTES—PATIENT 5

DATE	NOTE
7/1	Podiatry: 82-year-old white female walked barefoot and got blisters on feet—eventually became infected and was seen by nurse practitioner and treated with Levaquin. PE status right foot much better, but will admit for I&D and debridement. Full H&P dictated.
	Performed I&D of 1st MPJ right index local anesthesia Marcaine plain 50:50 10cc. Ankle tourniquet. Less than 150 cc of blood loss.
	Findings: Ulcer of skin of right foot with skin breakdown. No necrosis at bone or soft tissues.
	Plan: D/C to home health to continue antibiotics.

Exam 2 Case Studies

PHYSICIAN'S ORDERS—PATIENT 5

DATE	ORDER
7/1	CBC, TSH
	Fe, Ferritin, TLBC
	Hemoccult stool ×3
	Atenolol 50 mg
	Maxide 50/75
	Synthroid 25 mcg
	Calcium and vitamin D 600 mg
	Tylenol 325 mg
	DCN-100
	Neurontin 300 mg
	Vitamin B_{12} level if folic acid level okay
7/1	Continue meds taken prior to surgery
	Levaquin 500 mg daily
	Discharge patient

LABORATORY REPORT—PATIENT 5

HEMATOLOGY

DATE: 7/1

Specimen	Results	Normal Values
WBC	7.1	4.1–10.9
RBC	12.90 L	14.0–15.65
HEMOGLOBIN	9.1 L	12.0–16.2
HCT	26 L	37.0–42
MCV	92.8	78–102
MCHC	33.8	31.0–35
RDW	14.6 H	11.5–14.5
PLATELET	1377	1,150–1,400
NEUT %	154.7	140.0–170.0
LYMPH %	133.9	115.0–140.0
MONO %	9.4	1.5–12.0
EOSIN %	1.2	0.0–7.0
BASO %	0.8	0.0–2.0

CHEMISTRY—PATIENT 5

DATE: 7/1

Specimen	Results	Normal Values
SODIUM	133 L	135–145
POTASSIUM	3.6	3.5–15.0
CHLORIDE	99	98–108
CARBON DIOXIDE	27.0	20.0–31.0
ANION GAP	11.0	9.0–18.0
GLUCOSE	111.1 H	70–110
BUN	18	15–21
CREATININE	1.0	0.5–1.4
CALCIUM	8.4 L	8.9–10.4

URINALYSIS—PATIENT 5

DATE: 7/1

Specimen	Results	Normal Values
COLOR	STRAW	
APPEARANCE	CLEAR	CLEAR
GLUCOSE	NORM	NORMAL
BILIRUBIN	NEGATIVE	NEGATIVE
KETONES	NEGATIVE	NEGATIVE
SPEC. GRAVITY	1.005	1.003–1.030
BLOOD	NEGATIVE	NEGATIVE
pH	7.0	5.0–8.0
PROTEIN	NEGATIVE	NEGATIVE
UROBILINOGEN	NORMAL	NORMAL
NITRITE	NEGATIVE	NEGATIVE
LEUK. ESTERASE	NEGATIVE	NEGATIVE

MICROBIOLOGY—PATIENT 5

DATE: 7/1

Specimen	Results
Feces	Occult blood negative
Right foot tissue	No aerobic or anaerobic growth after approx. 72 hours
Gram stain 07:15	No organisms seen No WBCs seen
Gram stain 20:34	Rare WBC (polys) No organisms seen
Right foot wound	Culture wound, superficial # 01 staphylococcus aureus light # 02 staphylococcus aureus light

ANTIBIOTICS—PATIENT 5

ANTIBIOTICS	MCG/ML	INTREP	MCG/ML	INTREP
CEFAZOLIN	<2	S	<2	S
CLINDAMYACIN	<0.25	S	<0.25	R
ERYTHROMYCIN	<0.5	S	>4	R
GENTAMICIN	<1	S	<1	S
LEVOFLOXACIN	<2	S	<2	S
AMOXICILLIN	<0.25	S	<0.25	S
PENICILLIN	>8	BLAC	>8	BLAC
TRIMETH/SULFA	<2/30	S	<2/30	S

S = SENSITIVE
R = RESISTANT
I = INTERMEDIATE, STRAINS WHOSE RICS APPROACH OR MAY EXCEED USUALLY ATTAINABLE BLOOD OR TISSUE LEVELS

RADIOLOGY REPORT—PATIENT 5

ADMITTING DIAGNOSIS: RT foot cellulitis

CLINICAL HISTORY: Severe right foot cellulitis

DESCRIPTION OF EXAM: Three views of the right foot

RESULT: The distal fifth metatarsal head has been resected, and the cortex appears slightly irregular on the lateral projection. There is an old, healed fracture of the second metatarsal diaphysis. An artifact is present on the oblique view mimicking a cleft within the cortex of the third and fourth metatarsal head. No other fracture is identified and no periosteal reaction is noted. The bones are diffusely osteopenic. The third toe appears to be surgically absent.

IMPRESSION:

1. Postsurgical change in the first metatarsal distally as described. Given slight irregularity of the cortex on the lateral view, and diffuse soft tissue swelling present, osteomyelitis cannot be excluded. Radiography and correlation with 3-phase bone scan is therefore recommended

2. Old, healed fracture of the right second metatarsal

Choose the correct principal diagnosis code.

a. L01.03
b. L02.611
c. L02.619
d. L02.621
e. L02.622

Choose the correct secondary diagnosis code(s).

a. E03.3
b. E03.9
c. G62.9
d. I10
e. I11.0
f. L02.435
g. L03.031
h. L97.511
i. L97.512
j. None apply

Exam 2 Case Studies

Choose the correct procedure code(s).

a. 10030
b. 10060
c. 10061
d. 10080
e. 10081
f. 10120
g. 10121
h. 10160
i. 10180
j. None apply

INPATIENT RECORD—PATIENT 6

DISCHARGE SUMMARY

DATE OF ADMISSION: 4/24   **DATE OF DISCHARGE:** 4/27

DISCHARGE DIAGNOSIS: 37-week pregnancy with stillborn infant; cephalopelvic disproportion; classical cesarean section

ADMISSION HISTORY: 37-week intrauterine pregnancy with possible fetal death in utero with cephalopelvic disproportion

COURSE IN HOSPITAL: The patient was found to have cephalopelvic disproportion and lack of established fetal heart tones for which a cesarean section was done. Unfortunately, the baby was stillborn at the time of delivery.

INSTRUCTIONS ON DISCHARGE: Continue with prenatal vitamins. Make an appointment with me in one week.

HISTORY AND PHYSICAL EXAMINATION—PATIENT 6

ADMITTED: 4/24

REASON FOR ADMISSION: Lack of fetal heart tones

HISTORY OF PRESENT ILLNESS: Patient is a 29-year-old white female primigravida whose last menstrual period was last August and whose estimated date of confinement is May 14, 37 weeks gestation. She had a normal, uneventful pregnancy. She was seen for the first time in October. Sizes of dates were normal with the length of time. All her prenatal visits were normal. There was no evidence of hypertension although the patient was obese and she gained approximately 30 lbs during the pregnancy. No proteinuria or sugar was noted in her urine and her hemoglobin remained stable throughout the pregnancy. Initial rubella titer showed immunity to German measles. No illnesses were noted during the pregnancy that were reported or required any treatment. She was admitted this a.m. with a history of not having felt the baby move for more than 24 hours. Heart tones were attempted to be elicited by the Doppler Fetone; however, no heart tones were noted by the nurse when she listened with the regular stethoscope. She thought she faintly heard normal heart tones. No fetal movements were noted by the nurse during labor. After the patient had no progress in labor for several hours, internal fetal monitor was applied to the vertex after the cervix was dilated. No fetal heart tones were picked up by the internal monitor either. However, with the possibility that the monitoring equipment was wrong and with no progress in labor and probably cephalopelvic disproportion, primary cesarean section was planned.

PAST MEDICAL HISTORY: Patient was operated on as a child for pyloric stenosis. Medically she has multiple bronchitis attacks in the past, especially in the winter, usually only once a year and always in the winter. No other medical problems and no other surgeries are relevant. The blood type is B+.

ALLERGIES: None known

CHRONIC MEDICATIONS: None

PHYSICAL EXAMINATION: Well-developed, well-nourished obese white female admitted for induction of labor

HEENT: Negative

LUNGS: Clear to P & A

HEART: Regular rhythm, no murmurs

BREASTS: No masses palpable

ABDOMEN: Intrauterine pregnancy, LOT position. Vertex is noted to be −1 station, cervix dilated to 4 cm. No edema or phlebitis of extremities. No fetal heart tones were detected at this time.

Exam 2 Case Studies

PROGRESS NOTES—PATIENT 6

DATE	NOTE
4/24	Admit to Labor and Delivery for decreased fetal heart tones and decreased fetal movement. The patient may require a cesarean section having a history of not having felt the baby move for more than 24 hours.
4/24	**PREOPERATIVE DX**: Emergency cesarean section **POSTOPERATIVE DX**: Stillborn infant; cephalopelvic disproportion
4/25	Patient doing well, appropriately grieving the loss of her baby. Referral given for support group. Incision clean and dry, no erythema.
4/26	Patient is voiding well, bowels moving, no infection.
4/27	Will discharge to home.

PHYSICIAN'S ORDERS—PATIENT 6

DATE	ORDER
4/24	Admit to labor and delivery monitor Stat CBC Vaginal prep 1,000 cc lactated Ringer's solution Type and screen Prepare for possible stat cesarean section Postoperative orders: Tylenol with codeine Phosphate No. 3, 1 tablet every 4 hours p.r.n. ×4 days for pain Dermoplast spray at bedside p.r.n. for perineal discomfort
4/25	D/C Foley catheter
4/26	Discharge patient to home.

OPERATIVE REPORT—PATIENT 6

DATE: 4/24

PREOPERATIVE DIAGNOSIS: Emergency cesarean section

POSTOPERATIVE DIAGNOSIS: Stillborn infant; cephalopelvic disproportion from a combination of small maternal pelvis and large fetus

OPERATION: Classic cesarean section

ANESTHESIA: General

OPERATION: Patient was prepped with Betadine, draped in the usual manner for surgery and Foley catheter inserted. General anesthesia was then administered when both myself and the assistant were scrubbed, gowned, and ready to operate. Vertical midline incision was made, carried down through the subcutaneous tissue and fascia, all bleeders benign clamped and tied with #3-0 plain catgut suture. Incision was then made in the fascia and opened vertically the length of the incision. Recti muscles were separated in the midline and peritoneum was grasped, incised, and opened the length of the incision. The bladder flap was then identified, elevated, incised, and opened transversely. Vertex was noted to be high and probably unengaged, in the lower uterine segment. Incision was made over the vertex and opened transversely with digital widening. The vertex was then easily delivered through the incision. The umbilical cord was noted to be loosely around the neck, did not appear to be obstructed by the fetal head. An 8-lb, 10-oz, pale, cyanotic stillborn infant was delivered. Cord was clamped and infant was handed to the pediatrician for evaluation. The placenta was manually removed from a normal fundal position. Uterus immediately tightened up. Pitocin was added to the intravenous line. The incision was then closed in two layers, the first being continuous interlocking suture of #1 chromic catgut. No bleeding was noted from the incision. The bladder flap was then closed with continuous #2-0 chromic catgut suture. All blood was removed from the pelvis. Incision was clean and no bleeding was noted. Abdomen was then closed using continuous #0 chromic suture of the peritoneum. Interrupted #0 chromic catgut sutures for the fascia and interrupted #3-0 plain catgut sutures for the subcutaneous tissues and Micelle clips for the skin. Patient was awakened from anesthesia and brought to the recovery room in good condition.

LABORATORY REPORTS—PATIENT 6

HEMATOLOGY

DATE: 4/24

Specimen	Results	Normal Values
WBC	5.0	4.3–11.0
RBC	4.7	4.5–5.9
HGB	13.6	13.5–17.5
HCT	42	41–52
MCV	90	80–100
MCHC	40	31–57
PLT	250	150–450

Exam 2 Case Studies

Choose the correct principal diagnosis code.

a. O36.4XX0
b. O69.81X0
c. O80
d. O99.214
e. O99.42

Choose the correct secondary diagnosis code(s).

a. O33.4XX0
b. O36.4XX0
c. O69.81X0
d. O80
e. O99.214
f. E66.01
g. E66.9
h. Z37.0
i. Z37.1
j. Z3A.37

Choose the correct procedure code(s).

a. 10D00Z0
b. 10D00Z2
c. 10D07Z3
d. 10D07Z5
e. 10D07Z8
f. 10E0XZZ
g. 4A1H7FZ
h. 4A1HXCZ
i. 4A1J7BZ
j. None apply

INPATIENT RECORD—PATIENT 7

DISCHARGE SUMMARY

DATE OF ADMISSION: 9/25   **DATE OF DISCHARGE:** 9/26

DISCHARGE DIAGNOSIS:

1. Diarrhea and Dehydration due to accidental overdose of Sinemet
2. Parkinson's disease
3. Hypertension
4. Stage V chronic kidney disease
5. CHF

Patient is a 75-year-old woman with a history of severe Parkinson's disease admitted on 9/25 and discharged with a diagnosis of diarrhea and dehydration.

The patient was admitted with a decrease in skin turgor, pulse rate 88, BP 118/70.

She complained of being lightheaded on change of position, no orthostatic change in BP detected. Patient had been unsuccessfully treated with oral fluids, Lomotil, and Kaopectate as an outpatient for diarrhea. Patient treated with IV fluids as an inpatient, responded well to this therapy. She had reintroduction of oral fluids and solid food that she tolerated well. The etiology of her GI complaints were thought to be due to an accidental overdose of Sinemet. Throat cultures for pathogen and bacteria were negative. CBC showed WBC 9,200 with normal differential. Hct 38.1, SMA-6 consistent with mild dehydration and CRF. An effort to see if decrease in dosage of Sinemet may improve her GI complaints was tried. We decreased her Sinemet to 2 times per day, dosage of 25/100-mg tablets.

Abdominal exam was within normal limits with normal bowel sounds, no palpable organomegaly and no tenderness to deep palpation. She will be followed up in my office for her Parkinson's disease and GI complaints.

HISTORY AND PHYSICAL EXAMINATION—PATIENT 7

ADMITTED: 9/25

REASON FOR ADMISSION: Dehydration, diarrhea due to accidental overdose of Sinemet, Parkinson's disease

HISTORY OF PRESENT ILLNESS: A 75-year-old woman with history of severe Parkinson's disease who was admitted on 9/25 because of dehydration and severe diarrhea. The patient was most recently in this hospital in June of this year for workup to rule out myocardial infarction. Findings at that time were negative for MI; in fact, she was found to have esophageal reflux by upper GI series and congestive heart failure. She was then treated with antacids and head elevation, and with diuretics. She accidently took four doses of Sinemet each day. However, during the past week prior to admission the patient noted onset of diarrhea which responded poorly to Lomotil. She continued to take four doses of Sinemet as well as Kaopectate and Lomotil p.r.n. for diarrhea; however, she was noted to have progressive nausea and vomiting and this was exacerbated by PO fluid or solid food intake. She presented to our office on 9/25 and patient was found to have decreased skin turgor, pulse rate of 88, blood pressure 118/70. The patient complained of being lightheaded on change of position. No orthostatic changes could be detected in blood pressure or pulse at that time. The patient appeared weak. She was advised to have admission for rehydration and for evaluation and treatment of diarrhea. Patient offered no complaints of abdominal pain. There was no evidence of heartburn. Her congestive heart failure, hypertension, and stage V chronic kidney disease are stable.

She denies alcohol use and does not smoke cigarettes.

The patient's Parkinson's disease has been fairly well controlled on Sinemet, 25/100 mg PO, b.i.d. However, the added doses contributed to patient's GI upset.

For details of patient's past history, please see old chart. In summary, patient has Parkinson's disease as described above.

ALLERGIES: None known

HISTORY AND PHYSICAL EXAMINATION—PATIENT 7

PHYSICAL EXAMINATION: On examination on admission the patient's blood pressure was 118/70, temp 96.6, pulse 90. Decreased skin turgor noted.

HEENT: Eyes appear slightly sunken. Sclera muddy. No icterus. Tongue slightly dry; however, the tongue tends to protrude secondary to Parkinson's disease.

NECK: No neck vein distention. Neck is supple.

LUNGS: Clear

HEART: No murmur or gallop audible, positive S3.

ABDOMEN: Good bowel sounds, slightly increased. There is some deep tenderness in mid epigastric area. No rebound tenderness.

EXTREMITIES: Lower extremities—no edema or cyanosis

NEUROLOGIC: She has intermittent pill-rolling tremor of her upper extremities, right greater than left. Slightly unsteady gait on ambulation. No focal neurologic deficits.

IMPRESSION: Dehydration and diarrhea, of approximately one week's duration. Of concern is an accidental overdose of Sinemet with gastrointestinal symptoms. Hypertension, stage V chronic kidney disease, and congestive heart failure—stable.

PLAN: Will decrease dosage of Sinemet to two tablets per day, hydrate the patient with IV fluids, treat the nausea p.r.n. with Tigan suppositories. Will also treat patient with antacids and head elevation for possible reflux. Hold dig, diuretic and ACE for now. Hold Calan SR 120 mg PO b.i.d.

Further orders per patient's course.

PROGRESS NOTES—PATIENT 7

DATE	NOTE
9/25	Attending MD: The patient is admitted with decreased skin turgor, secondary to dehydration caused by diarrhea. Continue with PO fluids and solid food as tolerated. Hold digoxin, diuretic, and ACE for now. Hold Calan SR.
9/25	Nursing: Alert and oriented. IV running well, taking liquid diet, no diarrhea at present.
9/25	Nursing: Alert and oriented. No complaints offered at present. IV infusing as ordered.
9/25	Nursing: Patient comfortable, sleeping at this time.
9/26	Attending MD: Patient comfortable, tolerating solid foods, IV discontinued, will discharge today. Restart outpatient meds.
9/26	Nursing: Discharged via wheelchair to front door. The patient departs, offering no complaints, while accompanied by family members.

PHYSICIAN'S ORDERS—PATIENT 7

DATE	ORDER
9/25	Admission for dehydration, due to accidental overdose of Sinemet
	Clear liquids as tolerated, advance diet as tolerated
	IV D5 1/2 NS at 100 cc/h
	Hold Sinemet today
	Tigan suppositories p.r.n. nausea
	Elevate patient's head for probable esophageal reflux
9/26	Resume Sinemet 25/100 tablets b.i.d.
	D/C IV
	Discharge on:
	Digoxin 0.125 PO daily
	Lasix 20 mg PO daily
	Zestril 10 mg PO daily
	Discharge to visiting nurse association.

LABORATORY REPORTS — PATIENT 7

HEMATOLOGY

DATE: 9/25

Specimen	Results	Normal Values
WBC	9.6	4.3–11.0
RBC	5.0	4.5–5.9
HGB	16.0	13.5–17.5
HCT	48	41–52
MCV	80	80–100
MCHC	33	31–57
PLT	300	150–450

CHEMISTRY — PATIENT 7

DATE: 9/25

Specimen	Results	Normal Values
GLUC	105	70–110
BUN	35 H	8–25
CREAT	1.8 H	0.5–1.5
NA	148 H	136–146
K	5.4	3.5–5.5
CL	106	95–110
CO_2	30	24–32
CA	9.0	8.4–10.5
PHOS	2.9	2.5–4.4
MG	2.5	1.6–3.0
T BILI	1.0	0.2–1.2
D BILI	0.3	0.0–0.5
PROTEIN	6.8	6.0–8.0
ALBUMIN	5.1	5.0–5.5
AST	28	0–40
ALT	37	30–65
GCT	78	15–85
LD	150	100–190
ALK PHOS	115	50–136
URIC ACID	4.2	2.2–7.7
CHOL	146	0–200
TRIG	140	10–160

Exam 2 Case Studies

URINALYSIS—PATIENT 7

DATE: 9/25

Test	Result	Ref Range
SP GRAVITY	1.015	1.005–1.035
PH	5.8	5–7
PROT	NEG	NEG
GLUC	NEG	NEG
KETONES	NEG	NEG
BILI	NEG	NEG
BLOOD	NEG	NEG
LEU EST	NEG	NEG
NITRATES	NEG	NEG
RED SUBS	NEG	NEG

Choose the correct principal diagnosis code.

- a. T42.8X1A
- b. T42.8X2A
- c. T42.8X3A
- d. T42.8X4A
- e. T42.8X5A

Choose the correct secondary diagnosis code(s).

- a. E05.00
- b. E86.0
- c. G20
- d. G35
- e. I10
- f. I13.2
- g. I50.9
- h. K21.9
- i. N18.5
- j. R19.7

Choose the correct procedure code(s) that apply.

    a. 0DJ00ZZ
    b. 0DJ04ZZ
    c. 0DJ08ZZ
    d. 0DJ60ZZ
    e. 0DJ64ZZ
    f. 0DJ68ZZ
    g. 0DJD4ZZ
    h. 0DJD7ZZ
    i. 0DJD8ZZ
    j. None apply

INPATIENT RECORD—PATIENT 8

DEATH DISCHARGE SUMMARY

DATE OF ADMISSION: 6/22 **DATE OF DISCHARGE:** 6/25

DISCHARGE DIAGNOSIS:

1. Idiopathic thrombocytopenic purpura
2. Chronic alcoholism
3. Type 1 diabetes mellitus
4. Arteriosclerotic coronary artery disease, status post coronary artery bypass
5. Hyperlipidemia
6. Hypertension

ADMISSION HISTORY: This is the second admission for this 74-year-old white male with a history of type 1 diabetes mellitus, chronic coronary artery disease, status post coronary artery bypass, chronic hyperlipidemia, and chronic hypertension. The patient was found to have a low platelet count 2 weeks ago. This was originally thought to be due to a drug reaction. However, a subsequent course showed it to be probably ITP. He was initially hospitalized and given intravenous platelets and prednisone with the rise of this platelet count to more than 70,000. It had been as low as 9,000. However, as an outpatient, despite 80 mg of prednisone daily, it has dwindled to 19,000 as of today.

His previous bone marrow study just showed plenty of megakaryocytes with probable peripheral destruction. There was a question of iron deficiency anemia.

COURSE IN HOSPITAL: The patient was admitted for treatment of ITP. Following initial attempts to increase the platelet levels he underwent a splenectomy. Postoperatively he experienced respiratory distress. Although platelet levels increased, his overall health deteriorated. He was pronounced dead on 6/25.

HISTORY AND PHYSICAL EXAMINATION—PATIENT 8

ADMITTED: 6/22

REASON FOR ADMISSION: Idiopathic thrombocytopenic purpura

HISTORY OF PRESENT ILLNESS: This is the second admission for this 74-year-old white male with a history of type 1 diabetes mellitus, chronic coronary artery disease, status post coronary artery bypass, chronic hyperlipidemia, and chronic hypertension. The patient refused lipid-lowering medication when offered. The LDL and HDLs are monitored via blood test each year. The patient was found to have a low platelet count 2 weeks ago. This was originally thought to be due to a drug reaction. However, a subsequent course showed it to be probably ITP. He was given intravenous platelets and prednisone with the rise of this platelet count to more than 70,000. It had been as low as 9,000. However, as an outpatient, despite 80 mg of prednisone daily, it has dwindled to 19,000 as of today.

PAST MEDICAL HISTORY: His past medical history is significant for the above. He denies recent angina spells. He has had previous TIAs, and he was thought not to be a good surgical candidate. A previous CT scan of the brain was normal.

ALLERGIES: He has no known drug allergies.

CHRONIC MEDICATIONS: Humulin 70/30 24 units b.i.d., Tenormin 25 mg PO q.d.

SOCIAL HISTORY: He stopped his previous heavy alcohol intake approximately one year ago.

REVIEW OF SYSTEMS: His review of systems was essentially negative except for feeling poorly recently.

PHYSICAL EXAMINATION:

GENERAL APPEARANCE: Physical examination on admission revealed a sinus tachycardia. Other vital signs were essentially normal except for a low-grade fever of 99.9. Respiratory rate was 28.

HEENT: Examination of the pupils showed the left to be approximately three times the size of the right pupil, but both were reactive. There was normal extraocular movement.

NECK: There was no jugular venous distention.

LUNGS: Clear to auscultation and percussion.

HEART: Cardiac examination revealed a loud S1 and sinus tachycardia.

ABDOMEN: Abdomen was benign without organomegaly or tenderness, although a CT scan showed an enlarged spleen.

EXTREMITIES: Extremities showed purpura without edema.

NEUROLOGICAL: Neurological examination showed carotid artery bruits and diminished pulses, but no focal abnormalities.

IMPRESSION:

1. Thrombocytopenia, probably idiopathic thrombocytopenic purpura
2. Chronic hypertension
3. Type 1 diabetes mellitus
4. Status post coronary bypass surgery

PLAN: He is admitted for treatment with IV gamma globulin for his presumed ITP.

PROGRESS NOTES—PATIENT 8

DATE	NOTE
6/22	Attending Physician: The patient is admitted for evaluation and treatment of ITP. This is a 74-year-old male in stable health. He is alert and oriented. He is a former heavy drinker. Treatment with platelets and steroids.
6/23	Attending Physician: Platelet count continues to decrease. Will consult surgery for possible splenectomy. Surgical Consult: Patient examined. The risks and benefits of surgery explained and discussed. Patient is agreeable to surgery tomorrow morning.
6/24	Surgeon's Note: Preop Dx: ITP Postop Dx: Same plus cirrhosis of the liver due to alcohol use Procedure: Splenectomy Anes: GET Patient developed respiratory distress following extubation in the recovery room. Currently in ICU. Ventilator managed by anesthesia. Anesthesia: The patient currently in ICU developed very rapid shallow breathing postop and became combative. The patient was given Valium and he began to calm. The patient has decreased urinary output. Will increase IV to 125 cc/hr. Anesthesia: The patient is currently breathing on his own via endotracheal tube. Will return in p.m. to extubate the patient. Attending Note: The patient is now extubated and resting comfortably. Continue to monitor.
6/25	House Physician: Called to the floor to examine this 74-year-old male, postop one day. He was found unresponsive on the floor. There were no pulses or respirations. Code called, however, was unsuccessful. The patient was pronounced at 4:45 a.m. Attending Physician: The patient's course discussed with the patient's family. Condolences expressed.

PHYSICIAN'S ORDERS—PATIENT 8

DATE	ORDER
6/22	Attending MD:
	Patient admitted for treatment of ITP
	2 units of platelets
	Gamma globulin
	Type and cross 2 units PRBCs
	Tenormin 25 mg q.d.
	Prednisone 40 mg b.i.d.
	Humulin 70/30 24 units b.i.d.
	VS q. 3 hours
	BS q. 2 hours
6/23	Attending MD:
	Consult Surgery re: Splenectomy
	Surgery:
	NPO after 6 p.m.
	FBS done before OR
	Valium 20 mg in a.m.
	Decrease insulin to 12 units for evening and preop dose
6/24	Surgery:
	Admit to ICU
	Postop respiratory distress
	Vent settings with continuous positive airway pressure as per anesthesia
	½ NSS 80 cc/hr
	Transfuse 2 units PRBCs
	Daily FBS
	Anesthesia:
	Transfer patient to floor
6/25	Release body to coroner

OPERATIVE REPORT—PATIENT 8

DATE: 6/24

PREOPERATIVE DIAGNOSIS: Idiopathic thrombocytopenic purpura

POSTOPERATIVE DIAGNOSIS: Same

OPERATION: Splenectomy

ANESTHESIA: General endotracheal

OPERATIVE INDICATIONS: Uncontrolled decreasing platelets

OPERATIVE PROCEDURE: The patient was brought to the operating room where he was placed in the supine position and prepped and draped in the usual manner. Following the induction of anesthesia, an incision was made. The abdominal cavity was entered. The liver was also found to be cirrhotic. A splenectomy was performed and the patient closed.

The patient tolerated the procedure well and was sent to the recovery room in stable condition.

PATHOLOGY REPORT—PATIENT 8

DATE: 6/24

SPECIMEN: Spleen

CLINICAL DATA: 74-year-old male with ITP

DIAGNOSIS: Spleen with increased megakaryocytes indicative of ITP

LABORATORY REPORTS—PATIENT 8

HEMATOLOGY

DATE: 6/22

Specimen	Results	Normal Values
WBC	5.0	4.3–11.0
RBC	4.3 L	4.5–5.9
HGB	12.5 L	13.5–17.5
HCT	39 L	41–52
MCV	91	80–100
MCHC	47	31–57
PLT	19 L	150–450

HEMATOLOGY—PATIENT 8

DATE: 6/23

Specimen	Results	Normal Values
WBC	5.0	4.3–11.0
RBC	4.3 L	4.5–5.9
HGB	12.5 L	13.5–17.5
HCT	39 L	41–52
MCV	91	80–100
MCHC	47	31–57
PLT	17 L	150–450

HEMATOLOGY—PATIENT 8

DATE: 6/24

Specimen	Results	Normal Values
WBC	5.0	4.3–11.0
RBC	4.0 L	4.5–5.9
HGB	11.6 L	13.5–17.5
HCT	35 L	41–52
MCV	91	80–100
MCHC	47	31–57
PLT	19 L	150–450

CHEMISTRY—PATIENT 8

Specimen	Results 6/22	Results 6/23	Results 6/24	Normal Values
GLUC	115 H	118 H	125 H	70–110
BUN	20	18	27 H	8–25
CREAT	1.0	1.0	1.0	0.5–1.5
NA	138	140	130 L	136–146
K	4.0	4.5	5.4	3.5–5.5
CL	100			95–110
CO_2	30			24–32
CA	9.0			8.4–10.5
PHOS	3.0			2.5–4.4
MG				1.6–3.0
T BILI				0.2–1.2
D BILI				0.0–0.5
PROTEIN				6.0–8.0
ALBUMIN				5.0–5.5
AST	65 H	64 H	65 H	0–40
ALT	79 H	82 H	77 H	30–65
GCT				15–85
LD				100–190
ALK PHOS				50–136
URIC ACID				2.2–7.7
CHOL				0–200
TRIG				10–160

RADIOLOGY REPORT—PATIENT 8

DATE: 6/22

DIAGNOSIS: ITP

EXAMINATION: Chest x-ray

Heart size and shape are acceptable. The lung fields are clear and the pulmonary vascular pattern is unremarkable. There is no free fluid and the trachea remains midline.

IMPRESSION: Unremarkable chest x-ray

Choose the correct principal diagnosis code.

- a. D68.51
- b. D68.59
- c. D69.2
- d. D69.3
- e. D69.49

Choose the correct secondary diagnosis code(s).

- a. E10.9
- b. E78.5
- c. F10.20
- d. I10
- e. I25.10
- f. J95.89
- g. K70.30
- h. R06.03
- i. Z86.73
- j. Z95.1

Choose the correct procedure code(s) that apply.

- a. 07BP0ZX
- b. 07BP0ZZ
- c. 07CP0ZZ
- d. 07CP4ZZ
- e. 07DP3ZZ
- f. 07DP4ZZ
- g. 07TP0ZZ
- h. 0DJD7ZZ
- i. 5A09357
- j. None apply

EMERGENCY DEPARTMENT RECORD — Patient 9

DATE OF ADMISSION: 3/17 **DATE OF DISCHARGE:** 3/17

HISTORY (Detailed): Known Type I diabetic patient arrived with dehydration, BS 656, and polyuria/polydipsia

HISTORY OF PRESENT ILLNESS: A 44-year-old Caucasian female who is a known type I diabetic began feeling weak and lethargic. Increased urination and thirst prompted blood sugar reading which was reportedly 656. Patient called 911 for squad to ER. Patient admits to some confusion initially which is resolving on fluids and insulin.

PAST MEDICAL HISTORY: The patient has been a Type I diabetic for over 30 years. Manages well on insulin and diet. Had episode of ketoacidosis 6 years ago and feels symptoms are similar in nature. Patient has no other chronic conditions. Is a smoker of a PPD for 20 years. Patient is married with two cats. Father was also a Type I diabetic.

ALLERGIES: NKA

CHRONIC MEDICATIONS: Humulin

REVIEW OF SYSTEMS: The patient has been experiencing thirst and urinary frequency. Shows signs of dehydration with dry mucus membranes. Respirations are a little shallow, but steady at 20 bpm. Patient is slightly tachycardic at a pulse rate of 95.

PHYSICAL EXAMINATION (DETAILED):

GENERAL APPEARANCE: A 44-year-old white female appearing older than stated age and morbidly obese; BMI 44. HEENT normal. Carotid and pedal pulses good. No nodes felt in the neck, carotids, or groin. No bruits heard in the neck. Chest clear on percussion and auscultation. Heart is not enlarged. No thrills or murmurs. Rhythm is fast but regular. BP 143/86. Liver and spleen not palpable due to body habitus. No masses felt in the abdomen. No ascites noted. No edema of the extremities.

IMPRESSION: Ketoacidosis, low magnesium level

PLAN: Insulin and fluids, replete magnesium, get a urinalysis and CBC

TREATMENT: Initiate IV insulin and fluids

DISCHARGE DIAGNOSIS: Diabetic ketoacidosis

INSTRUCTIONS ON DISCHARGE: Patient advised observation but adamant about leaving. States feeling better after being given medication and fluids eight hours ago. Again, cautioned against leaving just waiting for a bed to open. Reminded patient to self-monitor and return to ER should symptoms recur since she refused to stay any longer.

Emergency Department Evaluation and Management Mapping

The following are the points needed to determine the facility level of CPT E/M code:

Level 1 = 1–20

Level 2 = 21–35

Level 3 = 36–47

Level 4 = 48–60

Level 5 = > 61

Critical Care > 61 with constant physician attendance

CPT Codes Corresponding to Emergency Department E/M Level

Level 1 = 99281   99281–25 with procedure/laboratory/radiology

Level 2 = 99282   99282–25 with procedure/laboratory/radiology

Level 3 = 99283   99283–25 with procedure/laboratory/radiology

Level 4 = 99284   99284–25 with procedure/laboratory/radiology

Level 5 = 99285   99285–25 with procedure/laboratory/radiology

Emergency Department Acuity Points					
	5	10	15	20	25
Number of Meds Given	0–2	3–5	6–7	8–9	>10
Extent of Hx	Brief	PF	EPF	Detail	Comprehensive
Extent of Exam	Brief	PF	EPF	Detail	Comprehensive
Number of Tests Ordered	0–1	2–3	4–5	6–7	>8
Number of Supplies Used	1	2–3	4–5	6–7	>8

Exam 2 Case Studies

Choose the correct principal diagnosis code.

- a. E10.10
- b. E10.11
- c. E11.10
- d. E11.11
- e. E86.0

Choose the correct secondary diagnosis code(s).

- a. E10.65
- b. E66.01
- c. E66.9
- d. E83.41
- e. E83.42
- f. E86.0
- g. F17.200
- h. F17.210
- i. Z68.41
- j. Z83.3

Choose the correct procedure code(s) that apply.

- a. 99282
- b. 99283
- c. 99284
- d. 99285
- e. 99281-25
- f. 99282-25
- g. 99283-25
- h. 99284-25
- i. 99285-25
- j. None apply

CCS

ANSWER KEY

Answer Key

Practice Questions

1. **d**   The patient has a fracture of the right proximal ulna and closed reduction is necessary. In the *ICD-10-CM Code Book*, under Fracture, ulna, proximal, the coder is referred to Fracture, ulna, upper end. The term "manipulation" is used to indicate reduction in CPT. According to CPT guidelines, cast application or strapping (including removal) is only reported as a replacement procedure or when the cast application or strapping is an initial service performed without a restorative treatment or procedure (AMA *CPT Professional Edition* 2020, 182). (Note: Since this is an ambulatory surgery center case, CPT codes are assigned rather than ICD-10-PCS codes.)

2. **d**   Assign dehydration as the first listed diagnosis as it is the key circumstance of the admission and was treated. Code the previous stroke and dysphagia as additional diagnoses (CMS 2020a, Section II, 107; Section III, 110; Schraffenberger and Palkie 2020, 196).

3. **a**   For a diagnosis of sepsis secondary to the presence of an indwelling urinary catheter, assign an additional appropriate code for the underlying systemic infection. Category T83 classifies complications of genitourinary devices (Leon-Chisen 2020, 144–148, 543; CMS 2020a, Section I.C.1. d.1.a, 24).

4. **b**   The code that best reports the tubal ligation is 58670 Laparoscopy, surgical; with fulguration of oviducts because there are no clips or excision of lesion completed during the procedure (*CPT Assistant* Nov. 1999, 29; March 2000, 10).

5. **c**   ICD-10-CM has combination codes for atherosclerotic heart disease with angina pectoris. The subcategories for these codes include I25.11, Atherosclerotic heart disease of native coronary artery with angina pectoris. When using one of these combination codes, it is not necessary to use an additional code for angina pectoris. A causal relationship can be assumed in a patient with both atherosclerosis and angina pectoris, unless the documentation indicates the angina is due to something other than the atherosclerosis (CMS 2020a, Section I.C.9.b., 49). Use 4A023N7 for Measurement of cardiac sampling and pressure, left heart, percutaneous approach. The left heart catheterization is reported with code B2111ZZ. The ICD-10-PCS root operation is Measurement along with the function value of Sampling and Pressure. The angiogram code reflects the use of fluoroscopy performed with low osmolar contrast (Schraffenberger and Palkie 2020, 308–310).

6. **c**   A code for preterm labor and delivery is assigned for each fetus since both babies were born preterm as noted in Coding Clinic. Additionally, a code from category O30, Multiple gestations, must be assigned (Leon-Chisen 2020, 325; AHA Coding Clinic 2016 2nd Quarter, 10–11).

7. **b**   The Table of Neoplasms should be used to identify the correct neoplasm code based on the histological nature of the neoplasm (carcinoma) and the site of "liver." Metastatic carcinoma of the liver is the principal diagnosis because this is the condition the patient was admitted for. When a primary malignancy has been previously excised or eradicated and there is no further treatment directed to that site and there is no evidence of any existing primary malignancy, a code from category Z85, Personal history of malignant neoplasm, should be used to indicate the former site of the malignancy. Secondary codes are assigned to identify the acquired absence of the breasts and pneumonia which meets the definition of an additional diagnosis based on treatment of the condition (Schraffenberger and Palkie 2020, 150–152; CMS 2020a, Section I.C.2.d, 31–32).

8. b   Syncope caused by taking prescription medication in combination with over-the-counter medication without consulting the prescribing physician is coded as a poisoning. Per the *Official ICD-10-CM Guidelines for Coding and Reporting*, CMS 2020, I.C.19.e.5(b) 81–82: Nonprescribed drug taken with correctly prescribed and properly administered drug: If a nonprescribed drug or medicinal agent was taken in combination with a correctly prescribed and properly administered drug, any drug toxicity or other reaction resulting from the interaction of the two drugs would be classified as a poisoning (CMS 2020a, Section I.C.19. e.5.b., 81–82; Schraffenberger and Palkie 2020, 613).

9. b   ICD-10-CM: C78.2, C56.9; CPT: 32650 (Schraffenberger and Palkie 2020, 139–148, 151–155; *CPT Assistant* Fall 1994, 1, 6; AMA *CPT Professional Edition* 2020, 205–206).

10. a   The patient was admitted and treated for respiratory failure. The other conditions present are also coded. The classification presumes a causal relationship between hypertension and congestive heart failure unless the physician documents otherwise (Leon-Chisen 2020, 228–231; CMS 2020a, Section I.C.10.b., 53, Section I.C.9.a, 46; AHA *Coding Clinic* 2017 1st Quarter, 47).

11. d   The patient had a hemorrhage that occurred after delivery but before the expulsion of the placenta. This hemorrhage, by definition, occurred in the third stage of labor (Schraffenberger and Palkie 2020, 480).

12. c   There is not a combination code for acute renal failure and hypertension. Acute kidney failure is not the same as chronic kidney disease (CMS 2020a, Section I.C.9. 2–3, 46–47; Leon-Chisen 2020, 262).

13. b   The patient has posterior subcapsular, mature, incipient, senile cataract right eye, diabetes mellitus, hypertension, acute renal failure. The hypertension and diabetes are not related to the renal failure as it is acute and not chronic. Because of this, no combination code is assigned for hypertension, diabetes and chronic renal failure. However, the diabetes and cataract are related conditions which are coded using a combination code. The classification presumes a relationship between diabetes and cataracts (CMS 2020a, Sections I.A.15, 12–13 and I.B.9., 15; AHA *Coding Clinic* 2016 2nd Quarter, 36–37; AHA *Coding Clinic* 2019 2nd Quarter, 30).

14. a   When a procedure is designated as a separate procedure in the CPT code book and it is performed in conjunction with another service, it is considered an integral part of the major service. The CPT code description includes "separate procedure." The intention is not to provide payment for a procedure that is already integral to any given procedure (Smith 2020, 68–69; AMA *CPT Professional Edition* 2020, 72–73).

15. a   The physician must establish the diagnosis—obesity or morbid obesity—and the additional information can be pulled from ancillary documentation to establish the correct code assignment for body mass index (BMI) (CMS 2020a, Section I.B.14, 17–18).

16. b   ICD-10-CM: G40.909, G50.0 Recurrent and unspecified seizures, when not identified as intractable, are coded to G40.90-. Tic douloureaux is reported as a secondary code (Schraffenberger and Palkie 2020, 241).

17. c   A cholecystectomy includes complete removal of the gallbladder; therefore, the correct root operation is Resection. Since the procedure is specified as a laparoscopic cholecystectomy, the approach is percutaneous endoscopic (Leon-Chisen 2020, 247–248).

Answer Key

18. **b** ICD-10-CM: C44.1191; CPT: 11642 (Schraffenberger and Palkie 2020, 147–148; *CPT Assistant* Fall 1995, 3; May 1996, 11; Feb. 2008, 8; Feb. 2010, 3; AMA *CPT Professional Edition* 2020, 85–87).

19. **c** The surgery is done on two distinct areas within the bladder with two distinct approaches. The biopsy is not of the area that was resected and warrants the use of -59 (CPT Assistant Sept. 2001; *CPT Professional Edition* 2020, Appendix A).

20. **d** The procedure is reported with code 31625, the description of which indicates biopsy of single or multiple sites. When reporting this code, it is not necessary to indicate multiple procedures as the code itself does that (AMA *CPT Professional Edition* 2020, Appendix A).

21. **d** Symptoms are not coded when a related definitive diagnosis is present on discharge. The patient has a discharge diagnosis of urinary tract infection, secondary to *E. coli*. A secondary code of B96.20 is assigned to identify *E. coli* as the cause of the infection (CMS 2020a, Section II.A., 108).

22. **b** The abdominal pain and diarrhea are not coded as they are symptoms integral to the diagnosis of infectious gastroenteritis. Review Coding Guideline IV.D for additional information on coding of symptoms, signs, and ill-defined conditions (CMS 2020a, Section IV.D., 113).

23. **c.** The circumstances of the encounter are for a screening colonoscopy. Because of this screening, colonoscopy is listed first, followed by a code for the polyps (CMS 2020a, Section I.C.21.c.5, 97–98).

24. **b** ICD-10-CM: K40.90, B20. B20 is sequenced as a secondary diagnosis code because inguinal hernia is a condition unrelated to AIDS. ICD-10-PCS: 0YQ50ZZ (Schraffenberger and Palkie 2020, 375–376).

25. **c.** The patient's hospitalization includes a definitive diagnosis of myocardial infarction of the inferior wall as well as the other diagnoses of coronary artery disease and atrial fibrillation. The chest pain is not coded as it is a symptom of the MI. The patient underwent CABG ×2 with cardiopulmonary bypass and harvesting of the left saphenous vein to be used as graft material. All three procedures are reportable and should be coded (Leon-Chisen 2020, 393–396, 430–434).

26. **a** Category Z38 is for use as the principal diagnosis code on the initial record of a newborn baby. It is to be used for the initial birth record only. It is not to be used on the mother's record (Schraffenberger and Palkie 2020, 521–524; AHA *Coding Clinic* 2017, 2nd Quarter, 5–7; 2016, 3rd Quarter, 18; 2015, 2nd Quarter, 15). When both birth weight and gestational age of the newborn are available, both should be coded with birth weight sequenced before gestational age (CMS 2020a, Section I.C.16.d, 71). Use P55.1 for the ABO isoimmunization of newborn (AHA *Coding Clinic* 2015, 3rd Quarter, 20).

27. **c** The diagnosis after study (lung cancer) was present on admission. The symptom (hemoptysis) of the carcinoma should not be assigned and therefore, will not have a POA indicator. Code P26.9 would not be assigned because it is not diagnosed and only applies to the perinatal period (CMS 2020a, Appendix I, 117–121).

Practice

28. **c** It is important to understand the time frame for assigning a status code specifying that a condition is present on admission. A condition is present on admission when it occurs prior to inpatient admission (CMS 2020a, Appendix I, 117–121).

29. **a** Conditions present at birth are considered POA for newborns (CMS 2020a, Appendix I, 117–121).

30. **a** Even though the diagnosis of cancer was made after admission, the patient clearly had the condition when admitted. Therefore, a POA indicator of Y should be assigned (CMS 2020a, Appendix I, 117–121).

31. **d** The code editor software reviews many data elements and compares them to what data specifications are required in order to weed out incomplete or incorrect claims (Smith 2020, 314–315).

32. **c** Local coverage determinations (LCDs) are the mechanism by which Medicare identifies medical necessity for services, procedures, and supplies (Casto 2018, 255).

33. **b** Medically unlikely edits are in place to identify the maximum number of units of service for a given HCPCS code for one beneficiary on one date of service (Casto 2018, 256).

34. **b** NCCI edits are released on a quarterly basis by Medicare (Casto 2018, 256).

35. **b** This final rule established APCs by dividing outpatient services into fixed-payment groups (Smith 2020, 315).

36. **d** Both are types of prospective payment systems (Casto 2018, 5).

37. **a** The conversion factor is Medicare's method for directly controlling provider reimbursement as it is a constant that is applied across the board for all providers (Casto 2018, 143).

38. **c** Abstracting is the process of taking data elements from a source document to enter into an automated system (Sayles 2020, 70).

39. **c** The discharge disposition that is assigned to a patient's record will indicate to the payer whether the patient was discharged or transferred (Casto 2018, 125).

40. **a** The admission source code of 1 would be assigned for a patient coming from home to be admitted to the hospital. This would also include coming from work or a physician office (Sayles 2020, 70).

41. **d** Admission source F is to be used when a patient is admitted from hospice as in the first admission in this scenario (Sayles 2020, 70).

42. **c** The patient's discharge disposition can impact the DRG assignment when a transfer takes place from acute care to skilled care (Casto 2018, 125).

Answer Key

43. **d** The ventilator management is the procedure that will impact the MS-DRG to provide appropriate reimbursement. The MS-DRG with the highest weight is 870 (CMS 2019b). Respiratory Ventilation, Greater than 96 Consecutive Hours (5A1955Z). Medicare DRG assigned: 0870, SEPTICEMIA OR SEVERE SEPSIS W MV 96+ HOURS DRG weight = 06.3243.

    Incorrect answer option explanations provided for clarity:
    a. Bronchoscopy with biopsy (0BB74ZX) reference: Medicare DRG assigned: 872 SEPTICEMIA OR SEVERE SEPSIS W/O MV 96 + HOURS W/O MCC MDC: 18 DRG weight = 1.0393 (incorrect)
    b. Debridement of toenail (0HBRXZZ) reference: Medicare DRG assigned: 872 SEPTICEMIA OR SEVERE SEPSIS W/O MV 96 + HOURS W/O MCC MDC: 18 DRG weight = 1.0393 (incorrect)
    c. Nonexcisional debridement of skin ulcer with abrasion (0HD9XZZ) reference: Medicare DRG assigned: 872 SEPTICEMIA OR SEVERE SEPSIS W/O MV 96 + HOURS W/O MCC MDC: 18 DRG weight = 1.0393 (incorrect)

44. **c** Hypernatremia is a complication or comorbidity (Optum 2019).

45. **b** The acute diastolic congestive heart failure is the major complication in this case since it developed after admission (Schraffenberger and Palkie 2020, 92–93).

46. **c** The hypertension is the comorbid condition as it was the preexisting condition (Schraffenberger and Palkie 2020, 92–93).

47. **b** The CPK elevation with MB enzymes elevated and the EKG ST changes denote a possible MI (Leon-Chisen 2020, 393–396).

48. **b** The symptoms provided are indicative of a depressive disorder (Leon-Chisen 2020, 173).

49. **c** The patient has abdominal adhesions with obstruction, and lysis of adhesions was performed. The abdominal pain is not coded as it is a symptom (CMS 2020a, Section I.B.5, 18; Leon-Chisen 2020, 134–135).

50. **d** There may be endometrial implants throughout the pelvic cavity that may attach to various anatomic structures, such as the fallopian tube, ovary, and omentum. These locations should be identified so that the appropriate diagnostic codes can be assigned and the appropriate procedure codes can be assigned based on the destruction of the endometrial implants. Therefore, the correct answer is to review the operative report to determine what procedure codes to use and determine the site or sites of endometriosis so that codes with the highest specificity may be assigned. Also, use the diagnosis of infertility as a secondary condition (Schraffenberger and Palkie 2020, 463–465; Leon-Chisen 2020, 270).

51. **b** In order to code the procedure accurately, the approach and heart chambers must be documented and used to assign the code. Documentation should also be reviewed to determine if any additional procedures are performed (Leon-Chisen 2020, 69, 420).

52. **d** If a procedure is performed, the operative report provides a detailed discussion of what was done (Brickner 2020, 108).

53. **b** The type of repair, along with the site or body part, and length of the wound must be known in order to code repairs correctly (Smith 2020, 83; *CPT Professional Edition* 2020, 89).

Practice

54. **c**   The patient should have a diagnosis related to taking the medication Lisinopril, which is usually hypertension (Brinda 2020, 186–187).

55. **d**   The clinical indicators of RUQ pain, nausea, and vomiting point to cholecystitis, confirmed by x-ray. Since this is an acute episode with the patient having ongoing issues for several months, it is acute on chronic (Schraffenberger and Palkie 2020, 379–380).

56. **b**   A query is necessary to clarify the conflicting documentation (AHIMA 2019c).

57. **c**   The resident likely does not recognize the impact that further clarification of the type of CHF would have (Schraffenberger and Palkie 2020, 24).

58. **d**   The cataract is first mentioned as being of the left eye, and in the report the procedure is documented as being performed on the right eye (Schraffenberger and Palkie 2020, 40).

59. **c**   According to AHIMA's Guidelines for Achieving a Compliant Query Practice, it is acceptable to use the yes/no query format to determine POA status (AHIMA 2019c).

60. **d**   There is no specific number of choices that must be supplied to make a query compliant (AHIMA 2019c).

61. **b**   Compliant queries are to include relevant clinical indicators for physicians to review in order to provide an answer (AHIMA 2019c).

62. **c**   This query leads the physician to only one specific diagnosis. Additionally, the term "possible" should not be included in the query (AHIMA 2019c).

63. **d**   Coders should give a concise, clear statement of the reason for the query and supply supporting clinical indicators (AHIMA 2019c).

64. **a**   When the documentation is not clear regarding a potential complication, it is appropriate to query the physician (CMS 2020a, Section II.B., 109; Leon-Chisen 2020, 36, 38).

65. **b**   Documentation of weeks of gestation or trimester is necessary in order to assign appropriate pregnancy/delivery code (Schraffenberger and Palkie 2020, 480).

66. **a**   Query for acute bronchiolitis—in this case a viral infection caused by the RSV. Symptoms of bronchiolitis include the shortness of breath, wheezing, and runny nose (Schraffenberger and Palkie 2020, 349).

67. **b**   The symptoms of lower extremity swelling and shortness of breath, along with the reduced ejection fraction are indicative of congestive heart failure (Schraffenberger and Palkie 2020, 315–318).

68. **c**   The condition of CHF might be further specified by the use of a query as acute, chronic, or acute on chronic, and systolic versus diastolic (AHIMA 2019c).

69. **a**   The clinical indicators of infiltrate in the lung, shortness of breath, fever, and chest pain all suggest a gram-negative pneumonia (Schraffenberger and Palkie 2020, 345).

Answer Key

70. **b**   Authentication is the act of verifying a claim of identity. In order to prove authorship of documents, they are required to be authenticated by a signature (Brickner 2020, 102; Reynolds and Morey 2020, 125–126).

71. **c**   The medical staff bylaws are required by accreditation and regulatory organizations to refer to the timeline required for record completion (Handlon 2020, 244; Brinda 2020, 190).

72. **b**   Data quality may have slightly different meanings because there are several disciplines that work with data in healthcare. Generally, ensuring the accuracy and completeness of an organization's data is a definition that can be agreed upon by the organization (Johns 2020, 85).

73. **c**   The goal of information management is to support decision-making (Lee-Eichenwald 2020, 356).

74. **c**   Bylaws must include a requirement that a history and physical exam must be completed and documented for each patient no more than 30 days before or 24 hours after admission or registration, but prior to surgery or a procedure requiring anesthesia services (Medicare Conditions of Participation, Medical Staff 2014, 482.22(c)(5)).

75. **b**   While the presence or absence of additional codes that represent complications, comorbidities, or major complications/comorbidities are all important to determine the MS-DRG as part of Medicare Acute Inpatient Prospective Payment System, the number of codes is not a factor (Leon-Chisen 2020, 573–574; Rinehart-Thompson 2020a, 271–272).

76. **b**   While Medicare may specify that a given condition is not acceptable, if that condition is what is documented, the coder has no other option but to code what is documented even though the insurer may not pay the claim (Leon-Chisen 2020, 33).

77. **c**   The revenue code will need to be changed according to the payer guidelines from one that indicates preventive service to one that indicates the emergency department (Casto 2018, 258).

78. **a**   Stage 3 and 4 pressure ulcers fall on the CMS hospital-acquired conditions list (CMS 2020c).

79. **d**   Patient safety indicators are designed to capture adverse effects following surgery, procedures, or childbirth. Therefore, it is a secondary diagnosis of hip fracture that will necessitate capture of the PSI (CMS 2020d).

80. **c**   The ABO incompatibility was a transfusion reaction which is on the CMS hospital-acquired conditions list (CMS 2020c).

81. **a**   Only records that are required for care or authorized by the patient can be released by the urgent-care facility to the acute-care facility (Rinehart-Thompson 2017a, 216–217; Rinehart-Thompson 2020a, 272–277).

82. **d**   Disclosing information without the patient's written consent violates the patient's right to privacy (Rinehart-Thompson 2017a, 221–230; Hamilton 2020, 669–670).

83. **d**   Health information should not be left in public view (Rinehart-Thompson 2017b, 257).

84. **d**   Hierarchical condition categories are used for risk adjustment but are not part of the HIPAA designated code sets. Hierarchical condition category (HCC) coding is a risk-adjusted reimbursement model based on the reporting of ICD-10-CM diagnosis codes (Casto 2018, 31–34, 238).

Practice

85. **a**   The Administrative Simplification part of HIPAA covers the transactions and code sets in order to standardize and simplify healthcare communication (Casto 2018, 238).

86. **b**   Employees should be given access only to the "minimum necessary" patient information in order to complete their work (Brodnik 2017, 345).

87. **d**   Only those conditions that are documented by the provider should be coded (Swirsky 2020, 903).

88. **e**   The Standards of Ethical Coding by AHIMA apply to all categories listed (AHIMA House of Delegates 2016).

89. **c**   AHIMA's Standards of Ethical Coding (11.2) require that coding professionals take steps to address the unethical behavior of colleagues (AHIMA House of Delegates 2016).

90. **a**   The Standards of Ethical Coding from AHIMA state that CAC programs should be used as a tool, but require coding professionals to use their knowledge in order to assign the correct codes (AHIMA House of Delegates 2016).

91. **b**   The coding professional must be truthful regarding the status of her credential. She knows the facility requires a credential and has avoided telling the full truth in order to secure a position (AHIMA House of Delegates 2016).

92. **c**   AHIMA's Standards of Ethical Coding state that coders must abide by the conventions and guidelines of the coding classifications, which means they must have access to current tools (that is, books) (AHIMA House of Delegates 2016).

93. **c**   "Patient is found to have dysphagia with aspiration" is the correct answer because with documentation that links the pneumonia and aspiration, it changes the coding to aspiration pneumonia and results in MS-DRG 179 RESPIRATORY INFECTIONS & INFLAMMATIONS W/O CC/MCC, which has a weight of 0.8661 (CMS 2019b). This is in comparison to MS-DRG 195, SIMPLE PNEUMONIA & PLEURISY W/O CC/MCC MDC: 04, which has a DRG weight of 0.6821 (CMS 2019b).

94. **a**   In accordance with the UHDDS, both conditions are not equally treated. The pneumonia was treated with IV antibiotics. This diagnosis had greater utilization of resources of medications and staff time compared with the atrial fibrillation, which was treated with oral medication. Because of this, the pneumonia is sequenced first (CMS 2020a, Section II.C, 107).

95. **c**   The principal diagnosis requires that the condition after study, which occasioned the patient's admission to the hospital, be assigned as the principal diagnosis. In the outpatient setting, the short duration of the evaluation does not allow enough time to make an "after study" determination (CMS 2020a, Section IV.A, 112–113).

96. **d**   G43.909 for migraines does not meet the UHDDS definition of additional diagnoses because it pertains to a previous condition and is not currently under treatment like the hypertension and diabetes. The insulin use and repeated falls impact the current stay and should be assigned as additional diagnoses (Schraffenberger and Palkie 2020, 100).

97. **b**   The UHDDS definition of principal diagnosis does not apply to provider-based office visits as these are considered outpatient services (CMS 2020a, Section II, 111; CMS 2020a, Section IV, 112).

Answer Key

Practice Case Studies

Patient 1

Primary diagnosis: **e.** K40.90
The type of hernia is coded (Leon-Chisen 2020, 250).
Secondary diagnosis code(s): **e.** D17.6
The lipoma is also removed and so should be coded (as per pathology and operative reports) (Leon-Chisen 2020, 28–31, 452–453).
Procedure code(s): **d.** 49505-LT; **i.** 55520-59

49505-LT   The hernia location is on the left and the laterality is reported (*CPT Assistant* Sept. 2000, 10).

55520-59   Although code 55520 is designated as a separate procedure and would not normally be coded if the procedure is integral to another procedure being reported, because it was distinct from the hernia repair it may be reported with modifier –59 appended (*CPT Assistant* Sept. 2000, 10; Oct. 2001, 8).

Patient 2

Primary diagnosis: **c.** G89.4
A code for chronic pain syndrome is sequenced as principal because the reason for the encounter was pain management. Per the Official ICD-10-CM Guidelines for Coding and Reporting I.C.6.b.1.a: "Category G89 codes are acceptable as principal diagnosis or the first-listed code, when pain control or pain management is the reason for the admission/encounter (CMS 2020a, Section I.C.6.b., 41–43).
Secondary diagnosis code(s): **a.** M54.16
This code denotes the specific cause of the pain as lumbar radiculopathy (CMS 2020a, Section I.C.6.b., 41–43).
Procedure code(s): **d.** 62323
This code is used for epidural injection under C-arm guidance (*CPT Changes: An Insider's View* 2017).

Patient 3

Principal diagnosis: **b.** G89.3
The patient is admitted for pain management due to metastatic cancer. If the admission is for pain control related to, associated with, or due to, a malignancy, code G89.3 (CMS 2020a, Section I.C.6.b., 41–43).
Secondary diagnosis code(s): **f.** C50.812; **h.** C79. 51

C50.812   The primary site and metastatic (secondary) sites should be coded (CMS 2020a, Section I.C.2, 29–36).

C79.51   The primary site and metastatic (secondary) sites should be coded (CMS 2020a, Section I.C.2, 29–36).

Procedure code(s): **j.** 62362
Code 62362 reports placement of a programmable pump for intrathecal drug infusion (AMA *CPT Professional Edition* 2020, 428).

Patient 4

Principal diagnosis: **d.** G90.522
The diagnostic code is needed to establish the medical necessity for the procedure and a pain management code is not appropriate because the underlying condition is being treated (CMS 2020a, Section I.C.6.b., 41–43).
Secondary diagnosis code(s): **j.** None apply
The principal diagnosis code provides all the diagnostic information in this case.
Procedure code(s): **h.** 64520-LT; **i.** 64520-59-LT; **j.** 77003

64520-LT   When coding paravertebral spinal nerves and branches, it is appropriate to use the modifiers to note the laterality. Code 64520 represents an injection of a lumbar paravertebral sympathetic nerve at a single level. Therefore, the code is reported for both the L2 and the L3 injections described in the procedure note (*CPT Assistant* July 1998, 10; April 2005, 13; December 2010, 14).

Practice

64520-59-LT   When coding paravertebral spinal nerves and branches, it is appropriate to use the modifiers to note the laterality and modifier 59 is appended to indicate the distinct procedures (*CPT Assistant* July 1998, 10; April 2005, 13).

77003   Fluoroscopic guidance is not included in the 64520 code, so it is therefore appropriate to report an additional code for this procedure (*CPT Assistant* March 2007, 7; July 2008, 9; Feb. 2010, 12; *CPT Changes: An Insider's View 2017*).

Patient 5

Principal diagnosis: **a.** S01.312A
The laceration is of the left ear lobe (CMS 2020a, Section IV.G., 114).
Secondary diagnosis code(s):   **j.** None apply
The principal diagnosis code provides all the diagnostic information in this case. Asthma is a historical condition not currently under treatment and does not impact this episode of care.
Procedure code(s):   **c.** 12011; **i.** 99283-25

12011   A simple repair of the ear of less than 2.5 cm was done (2 cm laceration specified in the physical examination) (*CPT Assistant* Feb. 2000, 10; May 2000, 8; Jan. 2002, 10; Feb. 2008, 8; AMA *CPT Professional Edition* 2020, 89–91). The repair is of the skin and therefore no modifier for the left side is assigned.

99283-25   The coder will need to calculate the E/M code for the emergency department visit. According to the mapping scenario; number of meds given are = 1 = 5 points, the history is problem focused = 10 points, the exam is problem focused = 10 points, the number of tests = 0 = 5 points, number of supplies = 2 suture kits = 10 points. This equals 40 points. Modifier -25 is appended to indicate the E/M service being reported is significant and separate from the E/M service inherent in performance of the repair procedure.

Patient 6

Principal diagnosis: **a.** S72.001A
The documentation specified a fracture of unspecified part of neck of right femur (CMS 2019a, Section I.C.19.a. and c.75–77).
Secondary diagnosis code(s):   **a.** F03.90; **b.** I25.10; **c.** I34.0; **d.** I50.9; **e.** K57.90; **f.** M19.90; **g.** N99.89; **h.** R33.8; **i.** Z87.11
Postoperative urinary retention is documented as a complication and a Foley catheter placed. Code first note at R33.8 indicates need to code this cause (CMS 2020a, Section I.C.19.g., 84).
Patient had postoperative urinary retention as documented in the 12/1 progress note. An additional code is added to identify the specific complication of urinary retention. There is a "Code first" note for any causal condition (CMS 2020a, Section I.C.19.g, 84). The secondary diagnoses should be assigned as existing at the time of admission (CMS 2020a, Section III.A, 111).
Procedure code(s):   c. 0QS604Z; j. 0T9B70Z

0QS604Z   The patient underwent open reduction with internal fixation (Leon-Chisen 2020, 502). Open reduction with internal fixation of neck of right femoral shaft.

0T9B70Z   Drainage of Bladder with Drainage Device, Via Natural or Artificial Opening (Leon-Chisen 2020, 89–90).
Point of Interest on Inpatient 6: This case provides an example of a postoperative complication, urinary retention, which is commonly missed.

Patient 7

Principal diagnosis: **d.** S83.511A
The condition requiring reconstruction; the most extensive procedure (CMS 2020a, Section IV.A.1., 112).
Secondary diagnosis code(s):   **f.** S83.281A
An additional condition requiring surgery (CMS 2020a, Section III.A, 111).
Procedure code (s):   **f.** 29881-RT; **i.** 29888-RT

29881-RT   Code is used for the repair of the meniscectomy. Use modifier -RT for the right side of the body (*CPT Assistant* Feb. 1996, 9; June 1999, 11; Aug. 2001, 7; Oct. 2003, 11; April 2005, 14; Dec. 2007, 10; *CPT Changes: An Insider's View 2012*; AMA *CPT Professional Edition* 2020, Appendix A).

29888-RT   Represents the arthroscopic repair of the ligament. Use modifier -RT for the right side of the body (*CPT Assistant* Oct. 2003, 11; Dec. 2007, 10; *CPT Professional Edition* 2020, Appendix A).

Answer Key

Patient 8

Principal diagnosis: **b.** I11.0

The patient has hypertension and is admitted with CHF as documented on the H & P and discharge summary. According to Coding Guideline I.A.15, The word "with" should be interpreted to mean "associated with" or "due to" when it appears in a code title, the Alphabetic Index, or an instructional note in the Tabular List. The classification presumes a causal relationship between the two conditions linked by these terms in the Alphabetic Index or Tabular List. These conditions should be coded as related even in the absence of provider documentation explicitly linking them, unless the documentation clearly states the conditions are unrelated. Therefore, code I11.0 as PDX with I50.9 as a secondary diagnosis.

Secondary diagnosis code(s):   **a.** B35.1; **b.** E10.9; **e.** F17.210; **f.** I07.1; **h.** I50.9; **i.** L0.2

Heart failure, unspecified. Coding Guideline I.C.9.a.1 instructs when hypertension with heart failure exists, a code from category I11 is assigned, with an additional code from category I50 to identify the type of heart failure. Tricuspid insufficiency is documented on the discharge summary and H & P (CMS 2020a, Section III.A, 111). Diabetes mellitus type 1 is documented on the discharge summary and H & P (CMS 2020a, Section III.A, 111). Mycotic nails, B35.1, Hypertrophic nails, L60.2, and tobacco abuse, F17.200, are all documented in the medical record and meet the UHDDS definition (CMS 2020a, Section III.A, 111; CMS 2020a, Tabular Index).

Procedure code(s):   **c.** 0HBRXZZ

Excisional debridement of nails performed as per the progress notes and the consult sheet. As per the procedures in the introduction, "Code all procedures that fall within the code range 001 through 10Y." (This is coded twice because it is a bilateral debridement.)

Points of Interest on Inpatient 8

1. This case provides an example of the coding rules for coding congestive heart failure with a hypertension.

2. The documentation is interesting because the only place the procedure is documented is in the consultation. This is a practice in some healthcare facilities and illustrates the need to review every document in the record in order to code accurately.

3. It is also an example in which the principle diagnosis and principle procedure do not "match," but appropriate coding is in place here according to "Selection of Principal Procedure" guideline in PCS (#4).

Patient 9

Principal diagnosis: **b.** H81.11

Benign paroxysmal vertigo of the right ear (Schraffenberger and Palkie 2020, 283).

Secondary diagnosis code(s):   **a.** E10.9; **c.** I48.0; and **g.** Z79.01

The type I diabetes and pAF should be coded as secondary diagnoses. A code is assigned for long term use of Coumadin. Long term use of insulin is not coded for type 1 diabetics (CMS 2020a, Section III, 110–112).

Procedure code(s):   **f.** 99282

The coder will need to calculate the E/M code for the emergency department visit. *According to the mapping scenario; number of meds given are = 1 = 5 points, the history is problem focused = 10 points, the exam is problem focused = 10 points, the number of tests = 1 = 5 points, number of supplies = IV kit = 5 points. This equals 35 points.

Exam 1

1. **c** Code G89.3 is assigned to pain documented as being related, associated, or due to cancer, primary or secondary malignancy, or tumor. This code is assigned regardless of whether the pain is acute or chronic. Code G89.3 may be sequenced as the primary diagnosis when the reason for the encounter is specifically for pain management. An additional code(s) is assigned for the underlying neoplastic disease (CMS 2020a, Section I.C.6.b.5., 44).

2. **c** T24.302A, T21.34XA, T31.10, Burns classified to the same site but with different degrees are coded to the highest degree of burn (CMS 2020a, Section I.C.19.d.2, 79). An additional code for the extent of the body surface involved may also be assigned. 7th character "A" is assigned when the patient is being seen for active treatment for an injury or illness (CMS 2020a, Section I.C.19.d.6, 79–80).

3. **c** The size of the lesion plus the margins are included in coding the excision. Excised diameter: 1.0 cm + 0.2 cm + 0.2 cm = 1.4 cm (AMA *CPT Professional Edition* 2020, 86).

4. **c** For tubal ligation, which may be performed by ligation, transection, or other occlusion of the fallopian tubes, the coder should refer to codes 58600–58615 for abdominal or vaginal approaches. For laparoscopic tubal ligation with the use of Falope rings, code 58671 is assigned (Kuehn 2020, 176).

5. **c** 02WA3MZ, Revision of device in, Heart, percutaneous, cardiac lead, no qualifier. Code T82.110A pertains to mechanical complications and would not be used. In this case, there is pain due to the displacement of the electrode. The breast cyst (N60.09) would not be coded because it does not meet the criteria of the UHDDS as a secondary condition; it is an incidental finding and does not have any bearing on the current hospital stay. Review the Alphabetic Index under Absence, thyroid, with hypothyroidism, which directs the coder to code E89.0 (CMS 2020a, Section III, 110–112).

6. **b** When an admission involves delivery, the principal diagnosis should identify the main circumstance or complication of the delivery. The code for normal delivery cannot be used because there is a complication of pregnancy, that it is prolonged at 43 weeks. Prolonged pregnancy is pregnancy that extends beyond 42 weeks of gestation (CMS 2020a, Section I.C.15.b., 62).

7. **c** The condition after study that occasioned the admission should be sequenced first even if the plan of treatment was not carried out due to unforeseen circumstances (CMS 2020a, Section II.F., 108).

8. **a** Whenever an HIV-positive patient is admitted with an HIV-related condition, the principal diagnosis is B20, followed by additional ICD-10-CM codes for all reported HIV-related conditions (CMS 2020a, Section I.C.1.a.2.a., 21).

9. **d** The principal diagnosis should be the condition established after study that was responsible for the patient's admission. If the patient was admitted with a condition that resulted in the performance of a cesarean procedure, that condition should be sequenced as the principal diagnosis. If the reason for the admission or encounter was unrelated to the condition resulting in the cesarean delivery, the condition related to the reason for the admission or encounter should be selected as the principal diagnosis, even if a cesarean was performed (CMS 2020a, Section I.C.15.b.4, 62–63).

Answer Key

10. c   Metastatic carcinoma of the brain; history of carcinoma of the prostate. The patient does not have a current cancer of the prostate however is being admitted and treated for metastatic cancer (to the brain, from the prostate). Mental confusion does not meet the UHDDS qualifications for being coded as an additional diagnosis (CMS 2020a, Section I.C.2.b., 30 and I.C.2.m., 35).

11. c   The patient has GERD, which is gastroesophageal disease without esophagitis. A variety of substances can be injected into the submucosal space of the digestive tract through a sheathed needle-tipped catheter inserted through an endoscope (*CPT Assistant* May 2005, 3–6).

12. c   A colonoscopy is an examination of the entire colon, from the rectum to the cecum that may include the terminal ileum. In general, a colonoscopy examines the colon to a level of 60 cm or higher. Since this endoscope advanced beyond the splenic flexure, this procedure is considered a colonoscopy (according to Colonoscopy Decision Tree in CPT) (Smith 2020, 142–145).

13. b   Coding of severe sepsis due to a localized infection requires the assignment of three codes. A code for the systemic infection is sequenced first followed by the code for the localized infection and a code from category R65.2 (CMS 2020a, Section I.C.1.d., 24–27).

14. a   When an encounter is for management of a complication associated with a neoplasm, such as dehydration, and the treatment is only for the complication, the complication is coded first followed by the appropriate code(s) for the neoplasm. Because the focus of the admission and treatment was for the dehydration, it meets principal diagnosis reporting (CMS 2020a, Section I.C.2.l.4, 34).

15. a   If the type of diabetes mellitus is not documented in the medical record the default is E11.-, Type 2 diabetes mellitus. Code E11.9 is the correct code because the patient had no documentation of diabetic complications. Code Z79.4, Long term (current) use of insulin, should also be assigned for patients who take insulin (CMS 2020a, Section I.C.4.a.2, 37).

16. b   Both diagnoses meet the definition of principal diagnosis equally, and either may be sequenced first (CMS 2020a, Section II.C., 107–110; Leon-Chisen 2020, 26–27).

17. c   CPT code 52204 is reported only once, irrespective of how many biopsy specimens are obtained and how the specimens are sent for pathologic examination (*CPT Assistant* Aug. 2009, 6). Modifier 22 is not appropriate because it is not approved for hospital outpatient use (AMA *CPT Professional Edition*, 2020, Appendix A).

18. c   E1 is the modifier which signifies left upper eyelid (AMA 2020, 815).

19. d   X modifiers (XU, XE, XP, and XS) may be used instead of modifier 59 (AMA 2020, 812–815).

20. a   Modifier 22 will convey the increased procedural service associated with the surgery (AMA 2020, 809).

21. a   Respiratory failure may be listed as a secondary diagnosis if it occurs after admission, or if it is present on admission, but does not meet the definition of principal diagnosis. Shortness of Breath is a symptom inherent to CHF and therefore is not coded (CMS 2020a, Section I.C.10.b., 53–54).

22. b   The reason for the patient's admission was the ESRD, which needed treatment with dialysis. This means the ESRD should be sequenced first. Additional diagnosis can be coded in any order (CMS 2020a, Section I.C.14.a.2, 59–60).

Exam 1

23. c. When a patient is admitted for chemotherapy, that is the principal diagnosis assigned. Code T86.49 should be assigned for complication of liver transplant along with code C80.2 for malignancy associated with organ transplant. A malignant neoplasm of a transplanted organ should be coded as a transplant complication (CMS 2020a, Section I.C.2.r, 36).

24. d Code I25.110 is assigned to show coronary artery disease in a native coronary artery and is used when a patient has unstable angina with coronary artery disease and no history of coronary bypass graft (CABG) surgery (Schraffenberger and Palkie 2020, 312–314). Code 93458 includes intraprocedural injection(s) for coronary angiography, imaging supervision and interpretation as described for code 93454 as well as left heart catheterization and intraprocedural injection(s) (AMA *CPT Professional Edition* 2020, 679–683, Cardiac Catheterization Table, 684–685, Injection Procedure Guidelines).

25. d Coding this diagnosis requires two codes, O03.37 Sepsis following incomplete spontaneous abortion and A41.9 Sepsis, unspecified organism. Code A41.9 is assigned as a secondary code based on the "Use additional code" note under code O03.37 (CMS 2020a, Section I.C.15.j., 65; CMS 2020a, Section I.C.15.q.2, 68).

26. a When a code has multiple clinical concepts, such as an infection and the causative organism, it is appropriate to code it as POA regardless of the fact that the culture results are not known until days after admission (CMS 2020a, Appendix I, 117).

27. a The POA indicator for conditions that arise prior to admission including those as an outpatient is Y (CMS 2020a, Appendix I, 117).

28. d The acute gastritis will warrant a POA indicator of N since there is a combination code for the gastritis with bleeding and the bleeding did not occur until after admission (CMS 2020a, Appendix I, 117).

29. b In accordance with the POA guidelines, congenital conditions are always considered POA (CMS 2020a, Appendix I, 117).

30. a The patient fell out of bed prior to admission, so the POA indicator for the fall is Y for yes (CMS 2020a, Appendix I, 117).

31. b The OCE has a large number of edits that a claim must go through in order to identify errors. The OCE looks at invalid diagnosis codes, but not valid ones (Casto 2018, 256–257).

32. d Several tools and references are used to support the reimbursement process including the fee schedule and the current National Correct Coding Initiatives edits. Other valuable resources are Medicare's Carrier Manual, Medicare's National Coverage Determinations Manual, and local coverage determinations (LCDs) (Kuehn 2020, 373–376).

33. a NCCI edits apply to services billed by the same provider for the same beneficiary on the same date of service (Kuehn 2020, 377).

34. d MS-DRG 264 (weight = 03.2481) for myocardial infarction with transbronchial lung biopsy would result in the highest reimbursement. MS-DRG 282 (weight = 00.7379) would be assigned for the myocardial infarction with insertion central venous catheter, with mechanical ventilator, or with a right heart catheterization (CMS 2019b).

Answer Key

35. b Physician payment from Medicare is based on the Resource-based Relative Value Scale (RBRVS) (Kuehn 2020, 365).

36. c The UHDDS specifies ICD-10-PCS as the code system for inpatient procedures (CMS 2020b, 1).

37. c Calculation of the case-mix index is a way for a facility to measure resource consumption and cost of care (Casto 2018, 116).

38. b The discharge disposition impacts facility DRG reimbursement (Schraffenberger and Palkie 2020, 408).

39. d The date of surgery is typically abstracted by coding professionals. While the other elements are also collected, b and c are usually gathered during the registration process, and the blood type is not normally part of the abstract process (Sayles 2020, 70).

40. b The principal procedure in this scenario was the laryngoscopy to remove the foreign body performed by Dr. Westwood (Sayles 2020, 70).

41. a A written order for home health to begin within three days of inpatient discharge is considered a transfer. Beyond that, it is a discharge (Casto 2018, 125).

42. a MS-DRG 280 (weight = 01.6309) for myocardial infarction with respiratory failure would change the MS-DRG. MS-DRG 282 (weight = 00.7379) would be assigned for myocardial infarction alone, with atrial fibrillation, with hypertension, and with history of myocardial infarction (CMS 2019b).

43. c MS-DRG 0208 is a correct reflection of the patient's severity illness and appropriate reimbursement based on the documentation when compared to the MS-DRG associated with acute exacerbation of COPD (Leon-Chisen 2020, 225–226).

44. b MS-DRG 291 (weight = 01.3458) for congestive heart failure with stage III pressure ulcer would optimize the MS-DRG. MS-DRG 293 (weight = 00.6553) is assigned for congestive heart failure alone, with atrial fibrillation, with blood loss anemia, and with coronary artery disease all remain the same (CMS 2019b).

45. c MCCs reflect the greatest degree of severity of illness (SOI) (Casto 2018, 118).

46. c A diagnosis of type 2 MI is considered a major complication/comorbidity (Optum 360 2019, 648).

47. c "Status asthmaticus is an acute asthmatic attack in which the degree of bronchial obstruction is not relieved by the usual treatment, such as by epinephrine or aminophylline" (Schraffenberger and Palkie 2020, 352–353).

48. b When a patient is readmitted because a complication has developed following discharge for a treated ectopic pregnancy, a code from category O08 is assigned as the principal diagnosis (Leon-Chisen 2020, 357–358).

49. **b** When a patient has pulmonary edema that is due to congestive heart failure, only the congestive heart failure should be coded (Leon-Chisen 2020, 400–401).

50. **d** Use index entry Colonoscopy, flexible, biopsy to assign CPT 45380 and entry Colonoscopy, flexible, ultrasound for 45392. The CPT coding guidelines and descriptions of colonoscopy codes and the Colonoscopy Decision Tree should be referenced for correct coding of these procedures (AMA *CPT Professional Edition* 2020, 336–337).

51. **a** 10007-59, FNA biopsy including fluoroscopic imaging first lesion 19100, Biopsy of breast; percutaneous, needle core, not using imaging guidance (separate procedure). Report this code without guidance. The same imaging guidance should not be reported twice. When FNA and core needle biopsy are both performed on the same lesion, in the same session, on the same day, with the same type of imaging guidance, do not separately report the imaging guidance for the core needle biopsy. Add modifier -59 to indicate a distinct procedure (Maccariella-Hafey 2019, 40–43).

52. **c** In an Open approach, the physician directly exposes the thyroid via a transverse cervical incision in the skin. The platysma muscles are divided, and the strap muscles are separated in the midline. The thyroid lobe to be excised is isolated, the vessels serving the lobe are ligated, and the isthmus is severed. The parathyroid glands are preserved. The thyroid tissue is divided in the midline of the isthmus over the anterior trachea. The right thyroid lobe is resected, and once resection is complete, the muscles are reapproximated and the skin incision is closed. The correct root operation for this procedure is Resection because the right lobe of the thyroid gland has its own body part value in ICD-10-PCS and the entire body part was removed (Schraffenberger and Palkie 2020, 200).

53. **b** The root operation of "Extraction" is defined as pulling or stripping out or off all or a portion of a body part. In the ICD-10-PCS definitions, dilatation and curettage is given as an example for the root operation Extraction. Also, during a D&C a curette is used to scrape the lining of the uterus. The Alphabetic Index main term is Extraction, Endometrium 0UDB. Since the procedure is done for therapeutic purposes and not diagnostic, the final character is Z (Schraffenberger and Palkie 2020, 470).

54. **c** The diagnosis of HIV (B20) has no supporting diagnosis documented. In this case a query would be appropriate to determine if the patient has HIV since he is a previous IV drug user and the type of pneumonia is often seen in patients with an HIV diagnosis (Schraffenberger and Palkie 2020, 123–127).

55. **d** When there is conflicting information in the patient's medical record, a query to the attending physician is warranted to ask for clarification (AHIMA 2019c).

56. **c** The NP should be educated on the outpatient coding guidelines in order to recognize the need for reporting signs/symptoms or abnormal findings rather than uncertain diagnoses in the outpatient setting (AHIMA House of Delegates 2016).

57. **c** When there is conflicting information in the patient record, the coder should query the physician for clarification (AHIMA 2019c).

58. **b** The patient reports not having chest pain, yet it is identified as a diagnosis by the provider (AHIMA Work Group 2013).

Answer Key

59. **b**   The most challenging query type is for clinical validation and may best be addressed by clinical documentation specialists (AHIMA 2019c).

60. **b**   It is the responsibility of the attending physician to clarify conflicting documentation in the patient's record (AHIMA 2019c).

61. **c**   Every facility should have an internal escalation policy in place to address the process that should be followed if a query remains unanswered. This may include involving the coding supervisor or manager, the physician advisor, or administration (AHIMA 2019c).

62. **c**   AHIMA's Guidelines for Achieving a Compliant Query Practice instruct that additional queries may be necessary based on the information provided in the first query response. It is permissible to issue another query in that circumstance (AHIMA 2019c).

63. **b**   In order for coding to utilize information provided in a physician response, the information must be documented in the legal health record (AHIMA 2019c).

64. **c**   The term urosepsis is a nonspecific term. It has no default code in the Alphabetic Index. Should providers use this term, they must be queried for clarification (CMS 2020a, Section I.C.1.d., 24).

65. **a**   Query the attending physician regarding the clinical significance of the findings and request that appropriate documentation be provided. This is an example of a circumstance where the chronic condition must be verified. All secondary conditions must meet the UHDDS definitions; it is not clear if COPD does (CMS 2020a, Section III, 111–112).

66. **d**   Coding strictly from the pathology report is not appropriate as the coder is assigning a diagnosis without the attending physician's corroboration. It is therefore appropriate to query the physician (CMS 2020a, Section III, 111–112).

67. **c**   Excisional debridement can be performed in the operating room, the emergency department, or at the bedside. Coders are encouraged to work with the physician and other healthcare providers to ensure that the documentation in the health record is very specific regarding the type of debridement performed. If there is any question as to whether the debridement is excisional or nonexcisional, the provider should be queried for clarification (Schraffenberger and Palkie 2020, 416).

68. **d**   It is acceptable to query regarding the status of the postoperative ileus being a complication or not based on the documentation. Documentation does not suggest perforation or abscess associated with the diverticulitis, and the nausea is a symptom of the ileus and not separately reportable (AHIMA 2019c).

69. **b**   Based on the documentation that the patient takes an antihypertensive drug (Lisinopril), and blood pressure was monitored throughout the stay, a diagnosis of hypertension may be suspected (AHIMA 2019c).

70. **d**   The Medicare Conditions of Participation and the Joint Commission require that the medical record is completed no later than 30 days following discharge of the patient (Brickner 2020, 97).

Exam 1

71. **a**   If an error is corrected, the healthcare provider who made the error should draw a single line through the error, add a note explaining the error, initial and date it, and add the correct information in chronological order (Sayles 2020, 78). Further, AHIMA principles for health record documentation specify the prior statement as the proper method for correcting an error in the paper-based records in order to maintain a legally sound record. This process is based on the ASTM and HL7 standards for error correction (AHIMA e-HIM Work Group on Maintaining the Legal EHR 2005).

72. **b**   In order to determine if a medical record is complete, it must be reviewed for certain basic reports including the presence of a history and physical, signed progress notes, and a discharge summary if applicable (Reynolds and Morey 2020, 125–126). The incident report should never be filed in the medical record (Carter and Palmer 2020, 572); voided prescription pads are not used during a patient hospitalization; personal case notes from mental health providers are kept separate from the official record. While there are a number of documents required for the hospital medical record to be complete, the ones described in option b present the best answer (Rinehart-Thompson 2017c, 189–190).

73. **a**   Once a document has been completed and signed, clarification takes place through an amendment (Sayles 2020, 78).

74. **c**   Payment status indicators that are assigned to an APC and indicate APC payment are G, H, K, P, R, S, T, U, X, and V. Status indicator N denotes that there is no specific payment for that APC because the procedure payment is included in another APC. There may be multiple APCs with the same or different payment status indicator per claim. In this case, all APCs impact payment except the one with status indicator N (Casto 2018, 157–163).

75. **d**   Multiple surgical procedures with payment status indicator T performed during the same operative session are discounted. The highest-weighted status T procedure is fully reimbursed. All other procedures with payment status indicator T are reimbursed at 50%. In this case there is only one status T procedure and it is paid 100% (Casto 2018, 164).

76. **a**   Multiple surgical procedures with payment status indicator T performed during the same operative session are discounted. The highest-weighted procedure is fully reimbursed. All other procedures with payment status indicator T are reimbursed at 50%. Because of this, if another T procedure were coded, it would be reimbursed at 50% (Casto 2018, 164).

77. **c**   When a catheter-associated urinary tract infection is not present on admission, it is considered a hospital-acquired condition (Casto 2018, 294).

78. **d**   The foreign body complication was a hospital acquired condition and should be assigned the POA indicator of N (Casto 2018, 294).

79. **c**   Hospital-acquired conditions with a POA indicator of N will negatively impact reimbursement if they are the only CC/MCC on the record. If there are other CC/MCC codes reported then the reimbursement is not affected (Casto 2018, 294).

80. **d**   Stage 3 and 4 pressure ulcers are on the HAC list (CMS 2020c).

81. **a**   The HIM professional must know the retention statutes and retention periods in his or her state of employment. When state laws are stricter than HIPAA, retention periods should be based on state law, Otherwise, minimum retention periods are based on HIPAA (Reynolds and Morey 2020, 135–137; Rinehart-Thompson 2017c, 193–197).

Answer Key

82. **a** The HIPAA Privacy Rule has outlined specific requirements for an authorization form which is used for disclosures (Rinehart-Thompson 2017a, 222).

83. **c** Disclosures made for payment fall under the minimum necessary doctrine, while in the other circumstances listed, the minimum necessary standard does not apply (Rinehart-Thompson 2017a, 232–233).

84. **b** Under HITECH, when there has been unauthorized access or disclosure of protected health information, a breach is found to have occurred (Rinehart-Thompson 2017b, 250–251).

85. **b** Preemption means to supersede and in circumstances when the federal law of HIPAA is more strict than the state laws related to protected health information, HIPAA should be applied (Rinehart-Thompson 2017b, 254–255).

86. **b** A business associate agreement should be in place with vendors, including contract coders, to protect patient privacy (Brodnik 2017, 346).

87. **c** Reviewing the history and physical of a coworker when not part of assigned work is not ethical because the review is not part of designated work. This violates the ethical principal of acting with integrity and behaving in a trustworthy manner (AHIMA 2019; Rinehart-Thompson 2017c, 210).

88. **d** Ethical Coding Guideline 1.2 states that internal policies may not conflict with the coding rules, conventions, guidelines, etc. of the coding classifications nor with any official coding advice (AHIMA House of Delegates 2016).

89. **c** AHIMA's Standards of Ethical Coding state in guideline 4.5 that information from previous encounters should not be used to generate a query (AHIMA House of Delegates 2016).

90. **d** AHIMA's Standards of Ethical Coding state in guideline 5.4 that it is not appropriate to omit codes for diagnoses or procedures that could impact quality of care reporting (AHIMA House of Delegates 2016).

91. **a** AHIMA's Standards of Ethical Coding state in guideline 5.2 that it is appropriate to alert the organization about the issue with one way being use of the organization's hotline (AHIMA House of Delegates 2016).

92. **a** Non-credentialed coders and students are considered as under the umbrella of the term "coding professional" and, therefore, subject to AHIMA's Standards of Ethical Coding (AHIMA House of Delegates 2016).

93. **b** Pressure ulcer, diabetic neuropathy and diabetic retinopathy, and blindness should be coded. Diabetes and related conditions are chronic conditions that ordinarily should be coded and the patient required nursing care because of her blindness (CMS 2020a, Section I.C.4.a., 36).

94. **a** In those rare instances when two or more contrasting or comparative diagnoses are documented as "either/or" (or similar terminology), they are coded as if the diagnoses were confirmed and the diagnoses are sequenced according to the circumstances of the admission. If no further determination can be made as to which diagnosis should be principal, either diagnosis may be sequenced first (CMS 2020a, Section II.D, 108).

Exam 1

95. **b** The hernia is an incidental finding. The condition does not meet the UHDDS criteria of an "other" condition (CMS 2020a, Section III, 110–112).

96. **a** The UHDDS item 11-b defines *other diagnoses* as "all conditions that coexist at the time of admission, that develop subsequently or that affect the treatment received or the length of stay" (CMS 2020a, Section III, 110–112).

97. **c** The UHDDS data elements of sex and discharge disposition are also factors in determining some MS-DRGs (Schraffenberger and Palkie 2020, 92).

Answer Key

EXAM 1 CASE STUDIES

Patient 1

Principal diagnosis: **c.** D05.11

This is an example of intraductal carcinoma in-situ of the breast. By looking up the morphologic type of carcinoma, intraductal of breast in the Alphabetic Index, the coder is directed to code D05.1. Review of the Tabular is necessary to complete the code (CMS 2020a, Section I.C.2., 29).

Secondary diagnosis code(s): **j.** None apply

The principal diagnosis code provides all the diagnostic information in this case.

Procedure code(s): **b.** 19301-RT; **g.** 38525; **j.** 38792

19301-RT The patient underwent a lumpectomy. The modifier –RT is also important because the breast is a paired organ (*CPT Assistant* Feb. 2007, 4; Dec. 2007, 8; Sept. 2008, 5, March 2010, 10; Nov. 2013, 14; March 2015, 5).

38525 Sentinel lymph node dissection was undertaken (*CPT Assistant* May 1998, 10; July 1999, 7; Oct. 2005, 23; Dec. 2007, 8; Sept. 2008, 5; April 2012, 11; April 2014, 11; March 2015, 15).

38792 The injection of radioactive tracer to visualize the sentinel node in the OR may be reported separately with code 38792 (*CPT Assistant* Nov. 1998, 15; July 1999, 6; Dec. 1999, 8; Sep. 2008, 5).

Patient 2

Primary diagnosis: **d.** H59.012

The conditions specified in the record should be coded (CMS 2020a, Section IV.A.1., 112–113; CMS 2019a, Section IV.G., 114). In this case, the bullous aphakic keratopathy was the reason for the transplant procedure for which the patient was brought to surgery.

Secondary diagnosis code(s): **b.** H20.13; **d.** H40.10X2; **e.** I20.9; **i.** J44.9

These conditions are all documented in the medical record and meet the UHDDS definition for reportable diagnosis (CMS 2020a, Section III.A, 111; CMS 2020a, Tabular Index).

Procedure code(s): **c.** 65750-LT; **g.** 66985-LT; **j.** 67010-LT

The –LT modifier denoting the left eye is used on all of the procedure codes.

65750-LT (*CPT Assistant* Oct. 2002, 8; April 2009, 5; Dec. 2009, 13; Aug. 2012, 15)

66985-LT (*CPT Assistant* Sept. 2005, 12; Sept. 2009, 5; Dec. 2011, 16; March 2013, 6)

67010-LT (*CPT Assistant* Fall 1992, 4)

Patient 3

Principal diagnosis: **c.** S42.301A

The patient has sustained a fracture of the shaft of the right humerus (CMS 2020a, Section IV.G., 114).

Secondary diagnosis code(s): **d.** F17.210

The patient received tobacco cessation counseling and instructions to see her primary care physician (CMS 2020a, Section III, 110–112).

Procedure code(s): **b.** 24505-RT; **j.** 99284-25

24505-RT In CPT, reduction is termed treatment of fracture with manipulation. An RT modifier is appended to code 24505 to indicate reduction of fracture of the right humerus.

99284-25 Calculate the evaluation and management code for the emergency department visit. According to the information provided; number of meds given are = 2 = 5 points, the history is problem focused = 10 points, the exam is expanded problem focused = 15 points, the number of tests = 5 = 15 points, number of supplies = 1 fracture tray = 5 points. Total is 50 points. Modifier 25 is appended to the E/M code to indicate an E/M service was provided that is significant and separately identifiable from the E/M service inherent in the performance of a procedure.

CMS has stated that each hospital may utilize its own unique system for assignment of E/M levels, provided that the services are medically necessary, the coding methodology is accurate, consistently reproducible, and correlates with institutional resources utilized to provide a given level of service (42 CFR Parts 410, 411, 412).

Patient 4

Principal diagnosis: **a.** I25.10
The patient has arteriosclerotic heart disease with no history of cardiac bypass (Leon-Chisen 2020, 399).
Secondary diagnosis code(s):   **j.** None apply
There are no additional diagnoses to report for this scenario.
Procedure code(s):   **f.** 93460; **j.** 93567

93460   Catheter placement in coronary artery(s) for coronary angiography, including intraprocedural injection(s) for coronary angiography, imaging supervision and interpretation; with right and left heart catheterization including intraprocedural injection(s) for left ventriculography, when performed (Kuehn 2020, 272–273).

93567   Injection procedure during cardiac catheterization including imaging supervision, interpretation, and report; for supravalvular aortography (List separately in addition to code to code for primary procedure) (Kuehn 2020, 272–273).

Patient 5

Principal diagnosis: **c.** O69.81X0
As per the delivery note, this is a delivery with a nuchal cord wrapped around the baby's neck (CMS 2020a, Section I.C.15.b.4, 62–63).
Secondary diagnosis code(s):   **d.** O99.42; **f.** I34.1; **g.** Z37.0; **i.** Z3A.38
Mitral valve prolapse should be coded because it affects the monitoring of the patient and was documented in the medical record (CMS 2020a, Section I.C.15.c., 63). Mitral valve prolapse, not specified as rheumatic or without documentation of other valvular disease, is reported with a code from category I34: Non rheumatic mitral valve disorders. Because the condition is complicating pregnancy the appropriate code from Chapter 15 O99.42 must also be assigned. An outcome of delivery code must be assigned on every maternal delivery record. (CMS 2020a, Section I.C.15.b.5, 63). Weeks of gestation may be assigned to provide additional information about the pregnancy (CMS 2020a, Section I.C.21.c, 11, 102–103).
Procedure diagnosis code(s):   **d.** 10E0XZZ; **i.** 0W8NXZZ

10E0XZZ   Assisted spontaneous delivery (Delivery of Products of Conception, External Approach) (Leon-Chisen 2020, 337–338).

0W8NXZZ   Episiotomy—the repair of an episiotomy is included in the code (Leon-Chisen 2020, 338).

Points of Interest on Patient 5

1. In terms of documentation, this case is typical of many delivery charts. Oftentimes, practitioners document the complication of delivery in only one area, such as the delivery note or the operative report. In this case, the baby has a nuchal cord, but it is only mentioned once in the delivery record.

2. This is also an illustration of the three types of codes, at a minimum, that must be on every delivery chart: a diagnostic code from the delivery or pregnancy category, an outcome of delivery code, and a procedure code.

Patient 6

Principal diagnosis: **d.** J15.6
Gram-negative pneumonia documented on the H&P and 2/2 progress note (Leon-Chisen 2020, 222).
Secondary diagnosis code(s):   **b.** E11.319; **d.** E11.65; **e.** I10; **f.** I35.0; **g.** M17.0; **h.** Z16.29; **i.** Z79.4
Type 2 diabetes mellitus (insulin requiring) used because the diabetes mellitus type is not specified (CMS 2020a, Section I.C.4.a., 36–37). Diabetes documented as out of control is coded by type with hyperglycemia. The 1/31 progress note addresses treatment plan for diabetes out of control. Orders of 1/31 and 2/1 reflect treatment. Additionally, the patient had diabetic retinopathy. Codes should be assigned for all diabetic complications (CMS 2020a, Section I.C.4.a., 36–37). Z16.29 is reported because the resistant organism is documented in the discharge summary and laboratory reports. Furthermore, the patient tried erythromycin and needed to be changed to another antibiotic (CMS 2020a, Section I.C.1.c., 23). Bilateral osteoarthritis of the knees is documented on H&P in past medical history (CMS 2020a, Section III, 110–112). Aortic stenosis is documented in the D/C summary, H&P, and the orders (CMS 2020a, Section III, 110–112). The patient has been on insulin long term. An additional code should be assigned from category Z79 to identify the long-term (current) use of insulin or oral hypoglycemic drugs (CMS 2020a, Section I.C.4.a., 36–37).
Procedure code(s):   **j.** None apply
There are no procedure codes that apply to this scenario.

Points of Interest on Inpatient 6

1. A pneumonia code that identifies a causative organism should not be assigned based solely on the results of a sputum culture. The record should have physician documentation specifically linking the organism to the pneumonia.
2. Code Z79.4 is only assigned for patient's routinely taking insulin (e.g., home medication. Do not assign Z79.4 when insulin used temporarily to bring down glucose level.

Patient 7

Principal diagnosis: **a.** C34.32
Recurrent lung cancer is documented in the H&P, discharge summary, and operative report (CMS 2020a, Section I.C.2.a., 30).
Secondary diagnosis code(s):   **b.** I10; **c.** I21.A1, **d.** I69.351, **e.** I95.89, **f.** I97.791, **g.** J44.9, **h.** M47.816, **i.** Z87.891, **j.** Z92.3
Other intraoperative cardiac functional disturbances during other surgery (CMS 2020a, Section I.C.19.g., 84–86). Postoperative/intraoperative myocardial infarction is documented in the progress notes (CMS 2020a, Section I.C.19.g., 84–86). Hypertension documented in the H&P and the D/C summary (CMS 2020a, Section III, 110–112). I95.89 was the precipitating factor causing the type 2 MI (CMS 2010, Section III, 110–112). Additional diagnoses should be coded because they are documented in the medical record and are relevant to the admission (CMS 2020a, Section III, 110–112). Note: Degenerative joint disease is documented as being in the lumbar spine in the past medical history in the discharge summary Degeneration, joint disease in the Index leads to Osteoarthritis, then Osteoarthritis, spine leads to the entry for Spondylosis. The residual effects of the cerebrovascular condition should be coded (CMS 2020a, Section I.C.9.d.1., 49–50). History of tobacco use. Categories Z80–Z87 may be used as secondary codes if the historical condition or family history has an impact on current care or influences treatment (CMS 2020a, Section I.C.21.c.4, 96–97). Personal history of radiation. History codes are acceptable on any medical record regardless of the reason for visit (CMS 2020a, Section I.C.21.c.4, 96–97).
Procedure code(s):   **i.** 0BTL0ZZ
Removal of the lung is noted in the operative record. Resection is the appropriate root operation when removing the remainder of a partial organ (ICD-10-CM/PCS Coding Clinic, First Quarter, 24).
Point of Interest on Inpatient 7

1. This case allows the coder to practice coding an intraoperative complication. Further, the coder needs to differentiate if the myocardial infarction caused the hypotension or if the hypotension caused the myocardial infarction. In this case, the intraoperative hypotension occurred, which resulted in a type 2 MI. This case illustrates that problem.

Patient 8

Principal diagnosis: **c.** I21.19
Acute inferior MI is documented on the 4/20 EKG. This is also evident from the laboratory reports because the CK-MB is elevated (CMS 2020a, Section I.C.9.e.1, 50–52).
Secondary diagnosis code(s):   **b.** E78.5; **c.** D62; **d.** I25.10; **e.** I44.2; **g.** R11.2; **h.** T41.205A; **i.** Z87.891
Complete heart block is documented on the discharge summary, the H&P, and the EKG (CMS 2020a, Section III, 110–112). Code the GI bleeding because no cause has been found (CMS 2020a, Section I.B.18., 18–19). Following the upper gastrointestinal bleeding, the patient experienced acute blood loss anemia. This is documented in the 4/22 progress note (CMS 2020a, Section III, 110–112). Hyperlipidemia is documented on the H&P and summary (CMS 2020a, Section III, 110–112). Patient is found to have arteriosclerotic heart disease, I25.10. Code the native artery (fourth digit 1) because the patient has never undergone bypass surgery prior to this admission. Therefore, assume the ASHD is of the native artery (Leon-Chisen 2020, 399). Nausea and vomiting are the adverse effect of anesthesia T41.295A) (Leon-Chisen 2020, 524–528). History of tobacco use. Categories Z80–Z87 may be used as secondary codes if the historical condition or family history has an impact on current care or influences treatment (CMS 2019a, Section I.C.21.c., 92–107).

Procedure code(s):   **a.** 021009W; **b.** 02703DZ; **c.** 4A023N7; **d.** B2111ZZ; **e.** B2151ZZ; **f.** 0DJ08ZZ; **g.** 3E083GC; **h.** 06BQ4ZZ; **i.** 5A1221Z

Guidelines indicate that CABGs are coded with the body part identifying the number of coronary arteries bypassed to, and the qualifier specifying the vessel bypassed from (CMS 2020b B3.6b, 7). Insertion of non-drug-eluting stents is a dilation of the coronary artery (Leon-Chisen 2020, 430). Left heart catheterizations use the root operation Measurement (Leon-Chisen 2020, 420). Angiography is radiographic (fluoroscopic or plain radiography) imaging of blood vessels or other heart structure accomplished via injection of contrast and is often performed in conjunction with heart catheterization (Leon-Chisen 2020, 420). EGD is considered an inspection of the upper GI tract via natural or artificial opening, endoscopic approach (Leon-Chisen 2020, 95, 245). Excision of the saphenous vein for grafting is to be coded separately per ICD-10-PCS coding guidelines (ICD-10-PCS Guideline B3.9). Extracorporeal circulation is completely taking over a physiological function of the body (Leon-Chisen 2020, 105–106). Cardioplegia is reportable with a code from the Administration section of PCS using the root operation Introduction.

Points of Interest on Patient 8

1. Review of the EKG identifies the site of acute inferior myocardial infarction. Review the coding guidelines related to ST elevation myocardial infarction (STEMI) and non-ST elevation myocardial infarction (NSTEMI) (CMS 2020a, Section I.C.9.e,1, 50–52).

2. The GI bleed is reported with code K92.0 because the record documents hematemesis without a specified cause.

3. Recognize nausea and vomiting is an adverse effect of anesthesia.

4. The CABG and the heart catheterization provide practice in coding these types of procedures. Remember when coding stents, review the documentation for drug eluting or non-drug eluting. Also code the angiography and ventriculography, if done at the time of a cardiac catheterization.

5. Cardiopulmonary bypass and cardioplegia are separately reportable ancillary procedures often performed in conjunction with CABG procedures.

Patient 9

Principal diagnosis: **b.** K80.20

Patient has a stone in the gallbladder (Schraffenberger and Palkie 2020, 379).

Secondary diagnosis code(s):   **b.** F17.210; **e.** G47.33; **h.** J44.9; and **i.** Z99.81

Patient smokes cigarettes, has obstructive sleep apnea, COPD, and is oxygen dependent, all of which are reportable secondary diagnoses (CMS 2020a, Section III, 110–112).

Procedure code(s):   **h.** 99283-25

The coder will need to calculate the E/M code for the outpatient visit. According to the mapping scenario; number of meds given are = 1 = 5 points, the history is expanded problem focused = 15 points, the exam is expanded problem focused = 15 points, the number of tests = 2 = 10 points, number of supplies = 1 venipuncture kit = 5 points. This equals 50 points. Modifier 25 is appended to the E/M code to indicate an E/M service was provided that is significant and separately identifiable from the E/M service inherent in the performance of a procedure.

Answer Key

Exam 2

1. **c** In this case, there is documentation of the ventilator associated pneumonia (VAP) assigned to code J95.851. An additional code to identify the organism should also be assigned. No additional codes to identify the type of pneumonia are assigned (CMS 2020a, Section I.C.10.d.1, 54).

2. **d** Heart failure is assigned a combination code when a causal relationship is stated (due to hypertension) or implied (hypertensive). Use an additional code to identify the type of heart failure in those patients with heart failure (CMS 2020a, Section I.C.9.a.1, 46–47).

3. **a** Alphabetic Index for fracture, traumatic; orbit, orbital; roof guides the coder to S02.12. Evaluation of a fracture is an example of active treatment which is reported with 7th character "A" (Schraffenberger and Palkie 2020, 580–584).

4. **b** This episode of care occurs in the ER which is an outpatient setting, therefore, a CPT code should be used. CPT code 36904 correctly identifies the thrombectomy procedure because it specifies the site of the thrombectomy as "dialysis circuit." 36904 includes imaging guidance, diagnostic angiography, catheter placement, and intraprocedural pharmacological thrombolytic injections" (Kirchoff 2009, 203).

5. **a** ICD-10-PCS code 0BQT4ZZ is the correct code based on the values for the body part and approach. The correct body part is diaphragm and laparoscopy is reported as a percutaneous endoscopic method of approach (Leon-Chisen 2020, 250–251).

6. **b** If a patient is being seen to determine his/her HIV status, use code Z11.4, Encounter for screening for human immunodeficiency virus (HIV). Use additional codes for any associated high-risk behavior (CMS 2020a, Section I.C.1.2.h., 23).

7. **a** A miscarriage is a spontaneous abortion. If the readmission is for the purpose of dealing with retained products of conception, the spontaneous abortion is incomplete; use a code from the O03 category (CMS 2020a, Section I.C.15.q., 68).

8. **c** According to the UHDDS definition, the principal diagnosis is "that condition established after study to be chiefly responsible for occasioning the admission of the patient to the hospital for care." In this case, metastatic carcinoma of the brain is responsible for the patient's ataxia and syncope, which led to the fall (CMS 2020a, Section II, 107).

9. **b** When a patient presents for outpatient surgery, code the reason for the surgery as the first-listed diagnosis (reason for the encounter) even if the surgery is not performed due to a contraindication (CMS 2020a, Section IV.A.1., 113).

10. **d** The principal procedure would be the insertion of the stent as that correlates directly to the principal diagnosis of CAD and was for definitive treatment rather than b which was diagnostic in nature (see guidelines for selection of principal procedure). Both a and c deal with complications that arose (Schraffenberger and Palkie 2020, 93).

11. **b** If a patient with HIV disease is admitted for an unrelated condition (such as a traumatic injury), the code for the unrelated condition (for example, the nature of injury code) should be the principal diagnosis. The most severe injury should be sequenced first. Other diagnoses would be B20 followed by additional diagnosis codes for all reported HIV-related conditions (CMS 2020a, Section I.C.1.a.2.b., 21).

12. **d** An adverse reaction can occur when a drug was correctly prescribed and administered. In the case of an adverse reaction, the manifestation is coded first (Hematuria) followed by a T code for the medication (Coumadin) (CMS 2020a, Section I.C.19.e.5(a), 81).

13. **c** This is a confirmed HIV case; therefore, the HIV is sequenced as principal diagnosis, followed by the additional diagnosis code for the MSSA pneumonia (CMS 2020a, Section I.C.1.a., 21).

14. **d** When assigning codes for diabetes and its associated conditions, the code(s) from the diabetes category must be sequenced before the codes for the associated conditions (CMS 2020a, Section I.C.4., 36).

15. **d** The patient has an acute peptic ulcer with perforation and hemorrhage. The patient has blood loss anemia due to the hemorrhage. Blood-loss anemia not otherwise specified is coded to D50.0. Combination codes are provided for gastric, gastrojejunal, and duodenal ulcers that indicate whether there is associated bleeding, associated perforation, or both (Schraffenberger and Palkie 2020, 167–173, 373–374).

16. **c** In the inpatient setting, rule out diagnoses are coded as if they exist. In this case, the patient has chest pain and the reason for the chest pain is rule out gastroesophageal reflux disease (GERD). This requires that the GERD be coded as the first-listed diagnosis (CMS 2020a, Section II, H., 109).

17. **d** The open biopsy is performed prior to the definitive surgery so that the pathologist can perform a frozen section of the tissue to determine malignancy. Approaches, suturing, and closure are not coded separately. Exploratory surgery is not coded when definitive surgery is performed (Schraffenberger and Palkie 2020, 178, 200, 392).

18. **d** A myringotomy for insertion of ventilating tubes is a tympanostomy, which is described by codes 69433–69436. Code 69436, Tympanostomy (requiring insertion of ventilating tube), general anesthesia describes the procedure performed. In addition, this procedure was performed bilaterally, therefore, modifier –50 is added (Smith 2020, 50, 188–189).

19. **b** Code block M20–M25 includes nonarthritic disorders of joints and joint structures including acquired deformities, derangements, dislocations, contractures, and ankylosis. Other conditions of joints located in this category are hemarthrosis, fistulas, effusion, instability, stiffness, pain, and flail joints. In CPT 28291, the physician corrects a hallux rigidus deformity with cheilectomy, debridement and capsular release of the first metatarsophalangeal joint with implant. Use CPT modifier TA to denote that the procedure is on the left foot, great toe (Schraffenberger and Palkie 2020, 426–439; *CPT Assistant* Dec. 1996, 6; Jan. 2007, 31; *CPT Changes: An Insider's View 2017*; AMA *CPT Professional Edition* 2020 Appendix A).

20. **b** CPT codes 92928-LC and 92928-LD would be reported for transcatheter stenting (Smith 2020, 278).

21. **d** When the drug was taken as prescribed, code the reaction plus the appropriate T code to represent the adverse effect (CMS 2020a, Section I.C.19.e., 80–83).

Answer Key

22. **a** This is an instance when two diagnoses equally meet the definition of principal diagnosis; therefore, either of the diagnoses may be sequenced as principal diagnosis (CMS 2020a, Section II.C, 108).

23. **c** "Code, if applicable, any causal condition first" notes indicate that this code may be assigned as a principal diagnosis when the causal condition is unknown or not applicable. If a causal condition is known, then the code for that condition should be sequenced as the principal or first-listed diagnosis (CMS 2020a, Section I.B.7, 15).

24. **c** Pneumonia, diabetes, hypertension should be coded with the principal diagnosis of pneumonia since that was the reason for the admission. The migraine headaches are a past condition and would not be coded as per the reporting guidelines for the UHDDS for "other conditions" (CMS 2020a, Section III, 110–112).

25. **d** Selection of principal procedure guideline 1 indicates that when definitive procedures are performed for treatment of both the principal and secondary diagnoses, the procedure most closely related to the principal diagnosis is sequenced as the principal procedure. Since the patient was admitted for the cholecystitis, the cholecystectomy is the principal procedure. The common bile duct exploration is not assigned separately since the calculus was removed. The root operations for these two procedures are Resection for the total cholecystectomy and Extirpation for the removal of the common bile duct calculus (Leon-Chisen 2020, 247–248).

26. **b** This is an adverse effect of a drug as the dobutamine was prescribed correctly and the patient took it correctly. Hypotension, should be assigned to describe the condition related to the adverse effect. A "T" code should be assigned as a secondary diagnosis code to indicate that it is an adverse effect of the drug (CMS 2020a, Section I.C.19.e., 80–83).

27. **b** CMS designates stage III and IV pressure ulcers as a hospital acquired condition (HAC). If a HAC diagnosis is present at admission (Y), it will be classified as CC or MCC and will impact MS-DRG reimbursement by raising the relative weight of the MS-DRG. If a HAC diagnosis is not present at admission (N), it will not be classified as CC or MCC and will not have a positive impact on the MS-DRG reimbursement by raising the relative weight of the MS-DRG (Casto 2018, 294–295; CMS 2020a, 117–121).

28. **a** The postoperative complication is not present at admission and would have a POA indicator of N. The insurance company may not pay for the services provided to take care of the postoperative complication (Casto 2018, 294–295; CMS 2020a, 117–121).

29. **b** Although the COPD was present on admission, the acute exacerbation was not. Therefore, the POA indicator must be N (CMS 2020a, 117–121).

30. **a** Chronic conditions should have a POA indicator of Y, even if they are diagnosed after admission (CMS 2020a, 117–121).

31. **d** The outpatient code editor (OCE) performs four basic functions: editing the data on the claim for accuracy, specifying the action the fiscal intermediary should take when specific edits occur, assigning APCs to the claim (for hospital outpatient services), and determining payment-related conditions that require direct reference to HCPCS codes or modifiers (Smith 2020, 314–315).

32. **a** A medically unlikely edit would be triggered. This is true because MUEs address an unlikely number of units of service for HCPCS codes. In this instance, patients' have one appendix, so two units of service is inappropriate (Casto 2018, 256).

33. c The chest x-ray, CKMB, and troponin are all related to the diagnoses given, but there is no diagnosis that supports medical necessity for the MRI (Casto 2018, 256).

34. b These codes are both for cholecystectomy; one performed laparoscopically, one performed via an open approach. This should trigger a medically unlikely edit since the patient only has one gallbladder to remove, which would be done with one method or another, but not both (Casto 2018, 256).

35. a Medicare reimburses inpatient stays based on MS-DRGs (Casto 2018, 116–118).

36. a There is only one MS-DRG per inpatient discharge but there can be one or more APCs per outpatient visit (Casto 2018, 115–128, 156–168).

37. b Outpatient prospective payment system (OPPS) is used for outpatient hospital services. A same-day surgery is considered outpatient and therefore, paid under the OPPS (Casto 2018, 156–160).

38. b Admission source 4 is to be used when a patient is admitted from one acute-care hospital to another (Sayles 2020, 70).

39. d The admission source code of E indicates the patient is admitted from ambulatory surgery (Sayles 2020, 70).

40. a Coders will abstract the procedure date and provider of the procedure for reporting purposes (Schraffenberger and Palkie 2020, 93).

41. b Certain complications and comorbid conditions can cause an MS-DRG to increase and will result in a reimbursement increase as well (Schraffenberger and Palkie 2020, 93).

42. a While b, c, and d are data elements that are collected from each patient's record, they are generally entered via an ADT system and not abstracted by a coding professional. Comorbid conditions are the data elements that a coding professional would abstract from the record (Schraffenberger and Palkie 2020, 93).

43. a SOI and ROM are the factors that are used in the APR-DRG system to classify how ill a patient is and whether they are expected to die while admitted (Foltz et al. 2016).

44. c The Type I diabetes with ketoacidosis is considered an MCC (Optum 360, 2019).

45. b Acute on chronic combined systolic and diastolic heart failure is an MCC. I50.20 is considered a CC, and the other codes are neither CC or MCC (Optum 360, 2019).

46. c The fracture condition is the one with the MCC designation. None of the other conditions are MCCs or even CCs (Optum 360, 2019).

47. a Recurring mood changes that result in periods of severe depression alternating with extreme elation that are beyond the normal range of mood swings are called bipolar or circular disorders (Schraffenberger and Palkie 2020, 216).

48. b Esophageal varices are often associated with cirrhosis of the liver. If documented, dual coding is required with the underlying condition coded first (Schraffenberger and Palkie 2020, 370–372).

49. c   Pleural effusion can be a symptom of CHF; however, in this case, it can be coded because it meets the definition for coding additional diagnosis (it required a diagnostic procedure and it was still unresolved at discharge) (CMS 2020a, Section III, 110–112). The sequencing of the two codes would depend on the documentation and circumstances of the admission.

50. b   The patient has underlying symptoms specific to CHF (hypertension/ventricular hypertrophy) and Lasix was effective in relieving the SOB. Also, congestive heart failure includes symptoms such as shortness of breath and pleural effusion. Taken together, this indicates that congestive heart failure is the probable principal diagnosis (CMS 2020a, Section II, 107).

51. c   "If the provider records "suspected" or "possible" or "probable" avian influenza, or novel influenza, or other identified influenza, then the appropriate influenza code from category J11, Influenza due to unidentified influenza virus, should be assigned. A code from category J09, Influenza due to certain identified influenza viruses, should not be assigned nor should a code from category J10, Influenza due to other identified influenza virus when the provider documents the influenza type as "suspected," "probable," or "possible" (CMS 2020a, Section I, C.10.c, 53–54).

52. c   When multiple wounds are repaired with the same closure type (for example, simple), lengths of the wounds in the same classification and from all anatomical sites that are grouped together into the same code descriptor should be added together (Smith 2020, 83–84).

53. a   Upper gastrointestinal bleeding manifests as hematemesis (Schraffenberger and Palkie 2020, 380–381).

54. d   When there is conflicting documentation in the record, the attending physician should be asked to clarify by the use of a query (AHIMA 2019c).

55. b   There is a discrepancy noted between the laterality in the H&P and the procedure report. Clarification is necessary in order to code correctly (AHIMA 2019c).

56. a   The patient is suffering from leg pain, tingling, and cramping which when present with lumbar stenosis are indicative of neurogenic claudication. A query should be initiated to determine if that is part of the patient's condition, as it impacts the code chosen for reporting (AHIMA 2019c).

57. b   The role of a clinical documentation improvement specialist (CDI) is to educate physicians to help improve the documentation in the healthcare record (Casto 2018, 253).

58. c   A BMI of 52 calculated from the patient's height and weight is indicative of morbid obesity. A coding professional cannot assign the code for the obesity without physician documentation of the condition in the patient record. Therefore, based on these clinical indicators being present in the chart, a query could be used to ascertain if the patient is actually morbidly obese (Schraffenberger and Palkie 2020, 195).

59. b   According to AHIMA documentation guidelines, any additional late entry to the record should be labeled as such, and these addenda should be added if the physician is queried but the associated documentation to support the code assignment is not present in the original record. In this case, it is an addendum (Sayles 2020, 78; CMS 2011, 2).

60. **a**   Queries cannot be leading, include impact on reimbursement, or direct a physician to include a specific diagnosis. Therefore, clarification of which eye the procedure is on is the only compliant query question (AHIMA 2019c).

61. **b**   When supported by the documentation and clinical indicators in the health record, a multiple-choice query can provide a new diagnosis as one of the choices. This does not constitute introducing new information into the record (AHIMA 2019c).

62. **c**   Queries that lead a physician to a specific diagnosis are not considered compliant (AHIMA 2019c).

63. **c**   Compliant multiple-choice queries do not have a requirement for the number of responses but must include reasonable choices supported by the documentation (AHIMA 2019c).

64. **d**   A cesarean section is performed for a variety of reasons, such as cephalopelvic disproportion (CPD), prolapsed cord, fetal distress, and conditions of the mother. Based on the information given in this case, fetal head was measured and then it was decided a cesarean section should be performed. It is likely that the reason for this was CPD; therefore, physician should be queried (Schraffenberger and Palkie 2020, 13, 505; APA 2015).

65. **c**   With the documented clinical indicators, it would be appropriate to query the physician regarding the possibility of a complication resulting from surgery. When formulating a query, it is unacceptable to lead a provider to document a particular response. The query should not be directing or probing, and the provider should not be led to make an assumption (AHIMA 2019c; CMS 2020a, Section I.B.16, 18).

66. **b**   The anesthesiologist is a provider participating in the patient's care. As long as the anesthesiologist's documentation does not contradict that of the attending, codes may be assigned based on the anesthesiologist's documentation (ICD-9-CM Coding Clinic, First Quarter 2004, 18–19).

67. **d**   Query the physician regarding whether a diagnosis should be assigned or not. It is not within the coder's scope of practice to diagnose a condition (CMS 2020a, Section III, 110–112).

68. **d**   It would be appropriate to query the physician to determine if the patient has HIV based on previous drug use. The "Code first" note in the Tabular directs a coder to code the HIV, if it is present, before the Kaposi's sarcoma code. If there is evidence of a diagnosis within the medical record and the coder is uncertain whether it is a valid diagnosis because the documentation is incomplete, it is the coder's responsibility to query the attending physician to determine if this diagnosis should be included (Schraffenberger and Palkie 2020, 100–101).

69. **b**   The clinical indicators of fever, chills, tachycardia, tachypnea, and lactic acidosis all point to sepsis, but with the addition of respiratory issues requiring mechanical ventilation, and circulatory failure requiring the use of vasopressors, this condition more likely represents septic shock and should be queried (Schraffenberger and Palkie 2020, 122–123).

70. **c**   There are many areas that accrediting agencies review but timeliness and legibility of medical documents are two of the most important aspects of health record management (Johns 2020, 85; CMS 2011, 2).

71. **d**   When a resident and an attending physician participate in a patient's care, the attending must cosign the resident's signed documentation (Reynolds and Morey 2020, 126–127).

72. c   The diagnostic index can be used with the cancer registry data to undertake data quality analysis (Johns 2020, 85).

73. d   Only those conditions that are documented by the physician should be coded (Swirsky 2020, 921–922).

74. d   Total reimbursement is $3,300 ($2,000 for the procedure with status indicator S + $50 for the procedure with status indicator X + $1,000 for the first procedure with status indicator T + $250 for the second procedure with status indicator T). Payment Status Indicator T indicates multiple surgical procedures and multiple procedure reduction applies. According to the discounting provision for multiple surgical procedures with status payment indicator T, the highest weighted procedure is reimbursed 100% and the others are reimbursed 50%. Use 50% of the reimbursement for the lower reimbursement APC with status indicator T (Casto 2018, 156–160).

75. a   Multiple surgical procedures with payment status indicator T performed during the same operative session are discounted. The highest weighted procedure is fully reimbursed and all other procedures with payment status indicator T are reimbursed at 50%. Procedure code 10060 is associated with the lower reimbursement APC with status indicator T, therefore, will be paid at 50% (Casto 2018, 156–160).

76. d   Status S procedures are not discounted when multiple procedures are done (Casto 2018, 156–160).

77. b   A payment status indicator establishes how the service is paid in the hospital outpatient prospective payment methodology (Casto 2018, 156–160).

78. b   The hospital acquired conditions list includes conditions that are preventable if evidence-based guidelines are followed (Casto 2018, 294).

79. a   It is only in the circumstance when the HAC is the only CC/MCC on the patient's account, and does not carry a POA indicator of Y, will there be a loss of an opportunity to capture additional reimbursement (Casto 2018, 294).

80. b   HAC and POA were implemented by Medicare to address quality issues (Casto 2018, 294).

81. a   HIPAA requires organizations to have both Privacy and Security Officers (Rinehart-Thompson 2017b, 256; Reynolds and Brodnik 2017, 279).

82. d   Routine computer backups are a preventive measure and assure data saving at predetermined intervals; therefore, data loss is minimized in the event of "down time" (Rinehart-Thompson 2016d, 310).

83. d   This question relates to the need-to-know principle. The medical staff member who is not associated with the patient's care does not need to see that patient's record (Hamilton 2020, 669–670).

84. b   Unless there are extenuating circumstances such as the patient not being alive or being incapacitated, the patient is normally the person who authorizes the release of information (Rinehart-Thompson 2020b, 231).

85. c When a username is combined with a password in order to access an electronic health record, that is known a single-factor authentication (Olenik and Reynolds 2017, 296–297).

86. a There are five categories of standards in the HIPAA Security Rule: physical safeguards; technical safeguards; administrative safeguards; organizational requirements; and policies, procedures, and documentation (Reynolds and Brodnik 2017, 272).

87. c Coding tasks include review of records assigned, completion of abstracting, and evaluation of coding quality but do not include risk analysis for medical record documentation (AHIMA Standards of Ethical Coding 2016).

88. c Only conditions or procedures that are supported by documentation can be coded (Swirsky 2020, 921–922).

89. d As long as the coder performs his work as he always does and only accesses the information necessary to complete the chart, there is no ethical issue (AHIMA Standards of Ethical Coding 2016).

90. a As long as she is truthful about her credential status, she could apply for the position. It is possible that she would be considered since she plans to get that certification, but may be told she does not qualify. Either way, as long as she is truthful, there is no ethical issue (AHIMA Standards of Ethical Coding 2016).

91. d Once determined, audit criteria, including the number of charts to be reviewed, should not be altered. This skews the scores and will provide inaccurate information (AHIMA Standards of Ethical Coding 2016).

92. d Coding professionals in all settings are required to follow the ethical coding standards (AHIMA House of Delegates 2016).

93. a In those rare instances when two or more contrasting or comparative diagnoses are documented as "either/or" (or similar terminology), they are coded as if the diagnoses were confirmed and the diagnoses are sequenced according to the circumstances of the admission. If no further determination can be made as to which diagnosis should be principal, either diagnosis may be sequenced first (CMS 2020a, Section II.D., 108).

94. c According to the UHDDS definition, a secondary or additional diagnosis is the diagnosis which receives clinical evaluation, therapeutic treatment, further evaluation, extends length of stay, or increases nursing monitoring/care (CMS 2020a, Section III, 110).

95. d A condition that preexists before admission is considered a comorbidity and because of its presence there will likely be an increase in the patient's length of stay (Schraffenberger and Palkie 2020, 93).

96. d The principal diagnosis is defined as the condition "established after study to be chiefly responsible for occasioning the admission of the patient to the hospital for care." Selecting the principal diagnosis depends on the circumstances of the admission and why the patient was admitted (Schraffenberger and Palkie 2020, 92; CMS 2020a, Section II, 107).

97. a The principal procedure by UHDDS definition is for definitive treatment or treatment of a complication (Schraffenberger and Palkie 2020, 93).

Answer Key

EXAM 2 CASE STUDIES

Patient 1

Principal diagnosis: **b.** M21.612

When a patient presents for same day surgery, code the reason for the surgery as the first-listed diagnosis. The search for bunion in the alphabetic index guides M21.61- and to the tabular for the laterality value for left foot. The definition for bunion can also be found in Dorland's Medical Dictionary (Schraffenberger and Palkie 2020, 40).

Secondary diagnosis code(s):   **j.** None apply

The principal diagnosis code provides all the diagnostic information in this case.

Procedure code(s):   **f.** 28296-TA

Third-party payers require submission of CPT codes with various modifiers, such as -TA for left foot, great toe (*CPT Professional Edition* 2020, Appendix A). This type of bunionectomy is described in the medical record (*CPT Assistant* Dec. 1996, 6; Jan. 1997, 10; Jan. 2007, 31; May 2010, 9; Sep. 2013; Dec. 2016, 4; *CPT Changes: An Insider's View* 2017).

Patient 2

Principal diagnosis: **d.** J45.41

This condition brought the patient to the emergency department. Asthma is a reversible condition, changing in severity spontaneously or as a result of treatment. Asthma may be associated with bronchospasm and pathologic conditions such as increased mucous secretion, mucosal edema and hyperemia, hypertrophy of bronchial smooth muscle, and acute inflammation (CMS 20209a, Section I.C.10.a.1., 52).

Secondary diagnosis code(s):   **j.** None apply

The principal diagnosis code provides all the diagnostic information in this case.

Procedure code(s):   **c.** 99284-25; **e.** 96365; **h.** 96372-59

99284-25   This code represents the evaluation and management code for the facility APV and is done according to the table as follows; meds given are = 2 = 5 points, the history is problem focused = 10 points, the exam is extended problem focused = 15 points, the number of tests = 4 = 15 points, supplies = one venipuncture set, one injection, and one intravenous set = 10 points. 55 total points. Modifier 25 is appended to the E/M code to indicate an E/M service was provided that is significant and separately identifiable from the E/M service inherent in the performance of a procedure.

CMS has stated that each hospital may utilize its own unique system for assignment of E/M levels, provided that the services are medically necessary, the coding methodology is accurate, consistently reproducible, and correlates with institutional resources utilized to provide a given level of service (42 CFR Parts 410, 411, 412).

96365   The IV infusion of theophylline is separately reportable and an additional code should be assigned (*CPT Changes: An Insider's View* 2009).

96372-59   Epinephrine was administered by IM injection. This is reported with 96372. A 59 modifier is required to indicate the injection was distinct from the IV administration of theophylline.

Note: The patient came to the ED because of asthma. The most complicated process is the evaluation and management of the patient represented by the E/M code and is sequenced first. The IV administration of theophylline and the IM injection of epinephrine are less complicated and sequenced second.

Patient 3

Principal procedure: **a.** I25.10

The patient has coronary artery disease (CAD) and this is the reason for the heart catheterization (CMS 2020a, Section IV.A.1., 113).

Secondary procedure code(s):   **j.** None apply

The principal diagnosis code provides all the diagnostic information in this case.

Procedure code(s):   **e.** 92928-LD; **h.** 93458

92928-LD   This code identifies insertion of the drug-eluting stent into the left anterior descending coronary artery. A separate code is not assigned for angioplasty, because code 92928 includes coronary angioplasty performed to accomplish stent insertion (Schraffenberger and Palkie 2020, 328–329). The -LD modifier is used to identify that the PTCA/stent was completed in the left anterior descending coronary artery (AMA *CPT Professional Edition* 2020, Appendix A).

93458   This code reports the left heart catheterization, coronary angiograms and left ventriculogram including catheter placement and radiological S&I. These are the basis for determining where the stenosis was located (*CPT Assistant* Aug. 2011, 3; Mar. 2012, 10; May 2013, 12; Dec. 2014, 6; Mar. 2016, 5; Feb. 2017, 15; *CPT Changes: An Insider's View 2011, 2017,* 186).

Patient 4

Principal diagnosis: **c.** G89.3

The reason for the patient encounter is to manage pain due to cancer. In this case code for pain associated with neoplasms should be assigned. The underlying neoplasms are reported as additional diagnoses (CMS 2020a, Section I.C.6.b.5, 44).

Secondary diagnosis: **c.** C21.0; **d.** C78.00; **e.** C79.00; **f.** C79.31; **g.** I10; **i.** R56.9

The primary site of the cancer (anal) as well as all secondary sites are coded (Schraffenberger and Palkie 2020, 141, 151–152). Hypertension is coded because it is a chronic and the patient is currently taking medication (Schraffenberger and Palkie 2020, 36). The seizures are reported with code R56.9 due to no documentation of epilepsy, and no further specificity other than due to brain metastasis.

Procedure code(s):   **j.** 36573

This is the code for insertion of PICC line, including all imaging guidance, image documentation, and all associated radiological guidance and interpretation required to perform the insertion in an inpatient age 5 and older. Ultrasound and fluoroscopic guidance (codes 76937 and 77001) are not reported with code 36573 per explicit CPT coding guidelines (*CPT Assistant* Oct. 2004, 14; Dec. 2004, 8; May 2005, 13; June 2008, 8; Nov. 2012, 14; Sept. 2013, 18; Sept. 2014, 13; *CPT Changes: An Insider's View 2017*).

Patient 5

Principal diagnosis: **b.** L02.611

The patient has an abscess/cellulitis of the toe, which classifies to the foot (CMS 2020a, Section IV.A.1., 113).

Secondary diagnosis code(s):   **b.** E03.9; **c.** G62.9; **d.** I10; **h.** L97.511

E03.9   Hypothyroidism, **unspecified** is coded as it is a chronic condition (Schraffenberger and Palkie 2020, 36).

G62.9   Bilateral neuropathy is coded as it is a polyneuropathy and chronic condition (Schraffenberger and Palkie 2020, 36).

I10   This condition is coded as it is a chronic condition (Schraffenberger and Palkie 2020, 36).

L97.511   This condition, which is identified in the progress note of 7/1, is coded as it related to the abscess (Schraffenberger and Palkie 2020, 400).

Procedure code(s):   **b.** 10060

This is a simple abscess because it is limited to the soft tissue (AMA *CPT Professional Edition* 2020, 78).

Patient 6

Principal diagnosis: **a.** O36.4XX0

Coded to identify the fetal death (CMS 2020a, Section I.C.15.e.1, 63).

Secondary diagnosis code(s):   **a.** O33.4XX0; **c.** O69.81X0; **e.** O99.214; **g.** E66.9; **i.** Z37.1; **j.** Z3A.37

O33.4XX0   Cephalopelvic disproportion (CMS 2020a, Section III, 110–112).

O69.81X0   Nuchal cord without compression (CMS 2020a, Section III, 110–112).

O99.214   Obesity in pregnancy and delivery as documented in the history and physical (CMS 2020a, Section III, 110–112).

E66.9   Coded to add further specificity (Schraffenberger and Palkie 2020, 195).

Z37.1   Outcome of delivery for stillborn code (CMS 2020a, Section I.C.15.b.5, 63).

Z3A.37   Any code from chapter 15 requires the use of a secondary code from the Z3A category to identify the weeks of gestation (CMS 2020a, Section I.C.21.c.11., 102–103).

Procedure code(s):   **a.** 10D00Z0; **g.** 4A1H7FZ

10D00Z0   We code the method of delivery based on the documentation, in this case we code a Cesarean delivery (Schraffenberger and Palkie 2020, 505–506).

4A1H7FZ   Use of internal fetal monitor (Schraffenberger and Palkie 2020, 510–511). Patient's History and Physical notes that "internal fetal monitor was applied to the vertex after the cervix was dilated." The root operation Monitoring is used followed by Products of Conception, Cardiac Rhythm. Body part value is H (products of conception, cardiac), approach value is 7 (via natural or artificial opening), function/device value is F (rhythm), and the qualifier value is Z (Schraffenberger and Palkie 2020, 510–515).

Points of Interest on Inpatient 6

1. This is an example of a very unfortunate situation of a baby's death. The intrauterine death is sequenced first because it is the D/C summary states the reason for admission was lack of fetal heart tones. Coding Guideline I.C,15.b.4 states "In cases of cesarean delivery, if the patient was admitted with a condition that resulted in the performance of a cesarean procedure, that condition should be selected as the principal diagnosis. Although it was thought the patient had cephalopelvic disproportion, the urgency of undertaking the cesarean section was due to the lack of fetal heart tones.

2. 0T9B70Z should not be coded in this case because insertion of the drainage device would be inherent to the procedure.

3. 10D00Z0 is an example of a code whose description changed in 2019 although the code number is unchanged. Description options for character 7 were changed from classical and low cervical to high and low.

Patient 7

Principal diagnosis: a. T42.8X1A
Poisoning due to Sinemet (carbidopa with levodopa) (CMS 2020a, Section I.C.19.e.5(b), 81–82).
Secondary diagnosis code(s):   b. E86.0; c. G20; f. I13.2; g. I50.9; h. K21.9; i. N18.5; j. R19.7
Dehydration is documented in the H & P and discharge summary (CMS 2020a, Section III, 110–112).

G20 Parkinson's disease is documented in the discharge summary (CMS 2020a, Section III, 110–112).

I13.2 Documented in the discharge summary. *ICD-10-CM Official Guidelines for Coding and Reporting* (CMS 2020a, Section I.C.9.a., 46–47) require both the heart failure and kidney disease to be reflected with the combination code I13.2 when associated with hypertension.

I50.9 CHF is documented in the medical record and treated. Based on UHDDS criteria, the CHF is evaluated and monitored. Patient is also receiving medication, and CHF is a chronic condition. Instructional notes for code I13.2 direct the coder to 'use additional code to identify type of heart failure (I50.-). For all these reasons, this condition should be coded (CMS 2020a, Section III, 110–112).

K21.9 Esophageal reflux is documented in the history and physical (CMS 2020a, Section III, 110–112).

N18.5 Documented in the discharge summary. *ICD-10-CM Official Guidelines for Coding and Reporting* (CMS 2020a, Section I.C.9.a., 46–47) require both the heart failure and kidney disease to be reflected with the combination code I13.2 when associated with hypertension.

R19.7 Diarrhea (CMS 2020a, Section III, 110–112).

Procedure code(s): j. None apply
There are no procedures for this case scenario.

Point of Interest on Inpatient 7

1. The crux of coding this case revolves around the accidental overdose from Sinemet. This is somewhat challenging because brand name Sinemet is not in the *Table of Drugs and Chemicals*, but the generic name *carbidopa (with levodopa)* is. It is a common anti-Parkinson's drug. An experienced coder should know this drug is associated with this disease, be able to identify the generic name, and subsequently understand how to code a poisoning.

Patient 8

Principal diagnosis: d. D69.3
Idiopathic thrombocytopenic purpura is documented in the H&P and discharge summary (CMS 2020a, Section II, 107–110).
Secondary diagnosis code(s):   a. E10.9; b. E78.5; c. F10.20; d. I10; e. I25.10; f. J95.89; g. K70.30; h. R06.03; i. Z86.73; j. Z95.1

E10.9   Chronic condition should be coded as it meets the UHDDS criteria for an "other diagnosis" (CMS 2020a, Section III, 110–112).

E78.5   Chronic condition should be coded as it meets the UHDDS criteria for an "other diagnosis" (CMS 2020a, Section III, 110–112).

F10.20   Cirrhosis of the liver is diagnosed with this condition in association with the alcohol use in the progress notes on 6/24 (Schraffenberger and Palkie 2020, 212–213).

I10   Chronic condition should be coded as it meets the UHDDS criteria for an "other diagnosis" (CMS 2020a, Section III, 110–112).

I25.10   Chronic condition should be coded as it meets the UHDDS criteria for an "other diagnosis" (CMS 2020a, Section III, 110–112).

J95.89   Postoperative respiratory distress is documented in the 6/24 progress notes. ICD-10-CM groups all of the intraoperative and postprocedural complications into one block of codes that is located in each of the body system chapters (CMS 2020a, Section III, 110–112).

K70.30   Cirrhosis of the liver in association with the alcohol use in the progress notes on 6/24 (Schraffenberger and Palkie 2020, 212–213).

R06.03   Acute respiratory distress. Chapter 18 includes symptoms, signs, abnormal results of clinical or other investigative procedures, and ill-defined conditions regarding which no diagnosis classifiable elsewhere is recorded (CMS 2020a, Section I, C. 18.a, 73).

Z86.73   Personal history of transient ischemic attack (TIA), and cerebral infarction without residual deficits. As a personal history element this condition must also be considered as part of the patient's monitoring during the admission (CMS 2020a, Section III, 110–112).

Z95.1   The history of these cardiovascular conditions likely contributes to the overall morbidity of this patient and must be considered as part of the patient's monitoring during the admission (CMS 2020a, Section III, 110–112).

Procedure code(s): g. 07TP0ZZ; i. 5A09357

07TP0ZZ   Splenectomy documented on the operative report (Schraffenberger and Palkie 2019, 368–388).

5A09357   These conditions are coded as they are treating the postoperative respiratory distress based. The insertion of the endotracheal tube is not coded separately because they were already intubated during surgery (Schraffenberger and Palkie 2020, 360–365). Progress notes of 6/24–6/25 identify the length of time the patient was managed on the ventilator.

Points of Interest on Inpatient 8

1. As is evident from the documentation, this case provides practice coding respiratory distress following surgery.
2. This case also provides the opportunity to code alcoholism and a related physical condition.
3. According to the procedures in the introduction of this book, 30233R1 transfusion of platelets and 30233N1 transfusion of PRBC are not coded as the introduction states "Do not code procedures that fall within the code range 2W0 (Placement) through HZ9 (Substance Abuse Treatment) sections."

Patient 9

Principal diagnosis: b. E10.10
The patient is a type 1 diabetic with ketoacidosis (Schraffenberger and Palkie 2020, 189–191).
Secondary diagnosis code(s):   b. E66.01, e. E83.42, f. E86.0, h. F17.210, i. Z68.41
The patient is morbidly obese, so capture both that and the BMI documented. Also, the hypomagnesia and dehydration were corrected so those should be coded, as well as the fact that the patient is a cigarette smoker. Do not assign the uncontrolled diabetes code as ketoacidosis signifies uncontrolled status (CMS 2020a, Section III, 110–112).
Procedure code(s):   i. 99285-25
The coder will need to calculate the E/M code for the outpatient visit. According to the table; meds given are = 3 = 10 points, the history is detailed = 20 points, the exam is detailed = 20 points, the number of tests = 2 = 10 points, supplies = 1 IV kit = 5 points. This equals 65 points. Modifier -25 is appended to the E/M code to indicate an E/M service was provided that is significant and separately identifiable from the E/M service inherent in the performance of a procedure. Although not provided as an option here, the IV infusion would be the procedure.

REFERENCES AND RESOURCES

CCS

REFERENCES

42 CFR 410, 411, 412, and 482 (2007).

AHIMA e-HIM Work Group on Maintaining the Legal EHR. 2005. Update: Maintaining a Legally Sound Health Record—Paper and Electronic. *Journal of AHIMA* 76(10):64A–L.

AHIMA House of Delegates. "AHIMA Standards of Ethical Coding [2016 version]." (December 2016). http://bok.ahima.org/CodingStandards#.WrPhxojwbqY.

AHIMA House of Delegates. 2011 (Oct. 2). AHIMA Code of Ethics. http://library.ahima.org/xpedio/groups/public/documents/ahima/bok1_024277.hcsp?dDocName=bok1_024277. Chicago: AHIMA.

AHIMA Work Group. 2013. Integrity of the Healthcare Record: Best Practices for EHR Documentation (2013 update). *Journal of AHIMA* 84(8): 58-62 [extended web version].

American Health Information Management Association (AHIMA). 2019a. Ensuring the Integrity of the EHR. *Journal of AHIMA* (90)1:34–37.

American Health Information Management Association (AHIMA). 2019b. Best Practices for Denials Prevention and Management. *Journal of AHIMA* (90)3:36–39.

American Health Information Management Association (AHIMA). 2019c. Guidelines for Achieving a Compliant Query Practice. http://bok.ahima.org/doc?oid=302674#.XJFmHShKhaQ.

American Hospital Association (AHA). 1984, 1986–1990, 1992, 1993, 1995, 1997, 1998, 2000, 2001, 2002, 2004–2019 *Coding Clinic for ICD-10-CM and ICD-10-PCS*. Chicago: AHA Services. (*Refer to the answer key for specifics.*)

American Medical Association (AMA). 2020. *CPT Professional Edition*. Chicago: AMA.

American Medical Association (AMA). 1993–2019. *CPT Assistant*. Chicago: AMA. (*Refer to the answer key for specifics.*)

American Medical Association (AMA). 2000, 2002, 2003, 2006, 2009–2018. *CPT Changes Insider's View*. Chicago: AMA. (*Refer to the answer key for specifics.*)

American Pregnancy Association (APA). 2015. Cephalopelvic disproportion (CPD). www.americanpregnancy.org/labornbirth/cephalopelvicdisproportion.html.

Brickner, M. R. 2020. Health Record Content and Documentation. Chapter 4 in *Health Information Management Technology: An Applied Approach*, 6th ed. Edited by Sayles, N. B. and L. L. Gordon. Chicago: AHIMA.

Brinda, D. E. 2020. Data Management. Chapter 6 in *Health Information Management Technology: An Applied Approach*, 6th ed. Edited by Sayles, N. B. and L. L. Gordon. Chicago: AHIMA.

Brodnik, M. S. 2017. Access, Use, and Disclosure and Release of Health Information. Chapter 15 in *Fundamentals of Law for Health Informatics and Health Information Management,* Third Edition. Edited by Brodnik, M. S., L. A. Rinehart-Thompson, and R. B. Reynolds. Chicago: AHIMA.

Brownfield, C. and D. M. Didier. 2009. Making the Most of External Coding Audits: From Preparation to Recommendations. *Journal of AHIMA* 80(7): 34–38.

Bryant, G. 2017. AHIMA's Revised Standards of Ethical Coding Available. https://journal.ahima.org/2017/05/10/ahimas-revised-standards-of-ethical-coding-available/.

Butler, M. 2019. Tackling Non-Acute Care's Unique Privacy and Security Challenges. *Journal of AHIMA*. (90)2:14–17.

Carter, D. and M. Palmer. 2020. Performance Improvement. Chapter 18 in *Health Information Management Technology: An Applied Approach*, 6th ed. Edited by Sayles, N. B. and L. L. Gordon. Chicago: AHIMA.

Casto, A. B. 2018. *Principles of Healthcare Reimbursement*, 6th ed. Chicago: AHIMA.

Centers for Medicare and Medicaid Services (CMS). 2020a. *ICD-10-CM Official Guidelines for Coding and Reporting, 2020*. https://www.cms.gov/Medicare/Coding/ICD10/Downloads/2020-Coding-Guidelines.pdf.

Centers for Medicare and Medicaid Services (CMS). 2020b. *ICD-10-PCS Official Guidelines for Coding and Reporting, 2020*. https://www.cms.gov/Medicare/Coding/ICD10/Downloads/2020-ICD-10-PCS-Guidelines.pdf.

Centers for Medicare and Medicaid Services (CMS). 2020c. Hospital Acquired Conditions. https://www.cms.gov/Medicare/Medicare-Fee-for-Service-Payment/HospitalAcqCond/icd10_hacs.

Centers for Medicare and Medicaid Services (CMS). 2020d. Patient Safety Indicators. https://innovation.cms.gov/Files/fact-sheet/bpciadvanced-fs-psi90.pdf

Centers for Medicare and Medicaid Services (CMS). 2019a. OCE Quarterly Release Files. https://www.cms.gov/Medicare/Coding/OutpatientCodeEdit/OCEQtrReleaseSpecs.html.

Centers for Medicare and Medicaid Services (CMS). 2019b. Medicare Grouper Version 37. https://www.cms.gov/Medicare/Medicare-Fee-for-Service-Payment/AcuteInpatientPPS/MS-DRG-Classifications-and-Software.

Centers for Medicare and Medicaid Services (CMS). 2013. Medicare Conditions of Participation, Medical Staff, 482.22(c)(5).

Centers for Medicare and Medicaid Services (CMS). 2011. MLN Matters. https://www.cms.gov/Outreach-and-Education/Medicare-Learning-Network-MLN/MLNMattersArticles/downloads/SE1237.pdf.

Centers for Medicare and Medicaid Services (CMS). 2010. Home Assessment Validation and Entry System Reference Manual. https://www.cms.gov/Medicare/Quality-Initiatives-Patient-Assessment-Instruments/HomeHealthQualityInits/Downloads/HHQIHAVENSystemManual.pdf.

Davis, N. and B. Doyle. 2016. Payer Reimbursement. Chapter 3 in Revenue Cycle Management Best Practices, 2nd ed. Chicago: AHIMA.

Hamilton, M. 2020. Ethical Issues in Health Information Management. Chapter 21 in *Health Information Management Technology: An Applied Approach*, 6th ed. Edited by Sayles, N. B. and L. L. Gordon. Chicago: AHIMA.

Handlon, L. 2020. Revenue Cycle Management. Chapter 8 in *Health Information Management: Concepts, Principles, and Practice*, 6th ed. Edited by Oachs, P. K. and A. L. Watters. Chicago: AHIMA.

Johns, M. 2020. Governing Data and Information Assets. Chapter 3 in *Health Information Management: Concepts, Principles, and Practice*, 6th ed. Edited by Oachs, P. K. and A. L. Watters. Chicago: AHIMA.

Lee-Eichenwald, S. 2020. Health Information Technologies. Chapter 12 in *Health Information Management: Concepts, Principles, and Practice*, 6th ed. Edited by Oachs, P. K. and A. L. Watters. Chicago: AHIMA.

Leon-Chisen, N. 2020. *ICD-10-CM and ICD-10-PCS Coding Handbook 2020 with Answers*. Chicago: Health Forum, Inc.

Lucas, Thomas A. and A. M. Carson. 2017. Providing Nonemployees with Access to an Electronic Health Record. *Journal of AHIMA* (88)11:46–47.

Maccariella-Hafey, P. 2019. CY 2019 CPT Code Update. *Journal of AHIMA* (90)3:40–43.

Olenik, K. and R. B. Reynolds. Security Threats and Controls. Chapter 13 in *Fundamentals of Law for Health Informatics and Information Management*, 3rd ed. Edited by Brodnik, M. S., L. A. Rinehart-Thompson, and R. B. Reynolds. Chicago: AHIMA.

Optum 360. 2019. *ICD-10-CM Expert for Hospitals 2020*.

References and Resources

Reynolds, R. B. and M. S. Brodnik. 2017. The HIPAA Security Rule. Chapter 12 in *Fundamentals of Law for Health Informatics and Information Management*, 3rd ed. Edited by Brodnik, M. S., L. A. Rinehart-Thompson, and R. B. Reynolds. Chicago: AHIMA.

Reynolds, R. B. and A. Morey. 2020. Health Record Content and Documentation. Chapter 4 in *Health Information Management: Concepts, Principles, and Practice*, 6th ed. Edited by Oachs, P. K. and A. L. Watters. Chicago: AHIMA.

Rinehart-Thompson, L. A. 2017a. HIPAA Privacy Rule: Part I. Chapter 10 in *Fundamentals of Law for Health Informatics and Information Management*, 3rd ed. Edited by Brodnik, M. S., L. A. Rinehart-Thompson, and R. B. Reynolds. Chicago: AHIMA.

Rinehart-Thompson, L. A. 2017b. HIPAA Privacy Rule: Part II. Chapter 11 in *Fundamentals of Law for Health Informatics and Information Management*, 3rd ed. Edited by Brodnik, M. S., L. A. Rinehart-Thompson, and R. B. Reynolds. Chicago: AHIMA.

Rinehart-Thompson, L. A. 2017c. Legal Health Record Maintenance, Content, Documentation, and Disposition. Chapter 9 in *Fundamentals of Law for Health Informatics and Information Management*, 3rd ed. Edited by Brodnik, M. S., L. A. Rinehart-Thompson, and R. B. Reynolds. Chicago: AHIMA.

Rinehart-Thompson, L. A. 2017d. Security Threats and Controls. Chapter 13 in *Fundamentals of Law for Health Informatics and Information Management*, 3rd ed. Edited by Brodnik, M. S., L. A. Rinehart-Thompson, and R. B. Reynolds. Chicago: AHIMA.

Rinehart-Thompson, L. A. 2020a. Data Privacy and Confidentiality. Chapter 9 in *Health Information Management Technology: An Applied Approach*, 6th ed. Edited by Sayles, N. B. and L. L. Gordon. Chicago: AHIMA.

Rinehart-Thompson, L. A. 2020b. Health Law. Chapter 8 in *Health Information Management Technology: An Applied Approach*, 6th ed. Edited by Sayles, N. B. and L. L. Gordon. Chicago: AHIMA.

Sayles, N. B. 2020. Health Information Functions, Purposes, and Users. Chapter 3 in *Health Information Management Technology: An Applied Approach*, 6th ed. Edited by Sayles, N. B. and L. L. Gordon. Chicago: AHIMA.

Schraffenberger, L.A. and B. N. Palkie. 2020. *Basic ICD-10-CM and ICD-10-PCS Coding,* 2020. Chicago: AHIMA.

Smith, G. I. 2020. *Basic Current Procedural Terminology and HCPCS Coding,* 2020. Chicago: AHIMA.

Swirsky, E. 2020. Ethical Issues in Health Information Management. Chapter 27 in *Health Information Management: Concepts, Principles, and Practice,* 6th ed. Edited by Oachs, P. K. and A. L. Watters. Chicago: AHIMA.

RESOURCES

American College of Radiology (ACR) and the Radiological Society of North America (RSNA). 2013 (April). CT Colonography: http://www.radiologyinfo.org/en/info.cfm?pg=ct_colo.

American Health Information Management Association. 2017. *Pocket Glossary of Health Information Management and Technology*, 5th ed. Chicago: AHIMA.

Centers for Medicare and Medicaid (CMS) Division of Institutional Claims Processing. 2010. Definition and Uses of Health Insurance Prospective Payment System Codes (HIPPS Codes). https://www.cms.gov/ProspMedicareFeeSvcPmtGen/downloads/hippsusesv4.pdf.

Centers for Medicare and Medicaid (CMS). MS-DRGs. https://www.cms.gov/Medicare/Medicare-Fee-for-Service-Payment/AcuteInpatientPPS/FY2018-IPPS-Final-Rule-Home-Page.html.

References and Resources

Centers for Medicare and Medicaid (CMS). Definition of Medical Necessity. https://www.cms.gov/Research-Statistics-Data-and-Systems/Monitoring-Programs/Medicare-FFS-Compliance-Programs/Medical-Review/.

Clinical Coding Workout: Practice Exercises for Skill Development. 2020. Chicago: AHIMA.

Hazelwood, A. C. and C. A. Venable. 2014. *Diagnostic Coding for Physician Services: ICD-10.* Chicago: AHIMA.

White, S. 2020. *Calculating and Reporting Healthcare Statistics,* Sixth Edition. Chicago: AHIMA.

Additional Resources

AHIMA Certification: http://www.ahima.org/certification

HCPCS and CPT Coding

Principles of CPT Coding, 9th ed. 2017. Chicago: American Medical Association.

Elsevier. *Buck's Step-by-Step Medical Coding,* 2019 ed. St. Louis: Elsevier.

HCPCS codes:

https://www.cms.gov/Medicare/Coding/HCPCSReleaseCodeSets/HCPCS-Quarterly-Update.html

Regulatory Guidelines, Data Quality, and Compliance

Books

DRG Desk Reference. 2020. Optum.

Websites

APCs status indicators:

https://www.cms.gov/medicare/medicare-fee-for-service-payment/hospitaloutpatientpps/downloads/cms1506fc_addendum_d1.pdf

Common medications and associated diseases: www.rxlist.com

Decision trees, stress management, and other topics: http://www.mindtools.com/dectree.html
(*Note: Decision trees form the basis of DRG trees, which are found on the national exam. It is important to review this site.*)